TOXIC... POCKET HANDBOOK

Michael J. Derelanko, Ph.D., D.A.B.T., F.A.T.S.

Department of Toxicology and Risk Assessment
Honeywell International Inc.
Morristown, New Jersey

CRC Press
Boca Raton   London   New York   Washington, D.C.

Library of Congress Cataloging-in-Publication Data

Cataloging information is available from the Library of Congress.

No claim to original U.S. Government works
International Standard Book Number 0-8493-0009-6
Printed in the United States of America 1 2 3 4 5 6 7 8 9 0
Printed on acid-free paper

ABOUT THE AUTHOR

Michael J. Derelanko, Ph.D., D.A.B.T., F.A.T.S., is Manager of Toxicology and Risk Assessment at Honeywell International Inc. (formerly AlliedSignal Inc.), Morristown, New Jersey. He received his B.S. degree from Saint Peter's College in 1973. He was a National Institute of Health predoctoral trainee in the Albert S. Gordon Laboratory of Experimental Hematology at New York University, receiving M.S. and Ph.D. degrees. He received the 1976 New York University Gladys Mateyko Award for Excellence in Biology. Following a two-year postdoctoral fellowship in pharmacology at Schering-Plough Corporation, he began his career in industrial toxicology in 1980 in the corporate toxicology laboratories of, what was at that time, Allied Chemical.

Dr. Derelanko is a Diplomate of the American Board of Toxicology and a Fellow of the Academy of Toxicological Sciences. He is a member of the Society of Toxicology, the Society for Experimental Biology and Medicine, and the honorary research society, Sigma Xi. He has served on the content advisory committee of the New Jersey Liberty Science Center, has chaired or been a member of industrial and government toxicology advisory committees, and serves on the speaker's bureau of the New Jersey Association for Biomedical Research.

Dr. Derelanko has authored more than 50 publications in experimental hematology, gastrointestinal pharmacology, and toxicology. He is co-editor along with Dr. Manfred Hollinger of the *CRC Handbook of Toxicology*. He has been actively involved in educating the public about toxicology, particularly at the middle school level, and has delivered invited lectures on this subject at national meetings. His current research interests include understanding the toxicity of aliphatic oximes.

Dedication

To all toxicologists in recognition of their efforts to protect human health and the environment.

PREFACE

Toxicologists rely on a large information base to design, conduct, and interpret toxicology studies and to perform risk assessments. Reference books such as the *CRC Handbook of Toxicology* kept in the toxicologist's office supply ready access to this information. However, reference books of this nature tend to be quite large in size and are not easily carried in a briefcase. This puts the traveling toxicologist at a loss when the need for toxicological reference information arises at meetings, conferences, or workshops, or when auditing studies at a contract laboratory. My goal was to produce a toxicological reference source in a convenient pocket-sized format that can supply needed toxicology reference information to the toxicologist traveling outside the lab or office.

Toxicologist's Pocket Handbook provides a small, easily carried reference source of basic toxicological information for toxicologists and other health and safety professionals. This book contains selected tables and figures from the larger *CRC Handbook of Toxicology* that I previously edited along with Dr. Mannfred Hollinger. These tables and figures contain the most frequently used toxicology reference information. An abbreviated glossary of commonly used toxicological terms is also included. As with the larger handbook, this book has been designed to allow basic reference information to be located quickly. Tables and figures have been placed in sections specific to various subspecialties of toxicology. A detailed table of contents contains a listing of all of the tables and figures contained in the book. As many of the tables and figures originally obtained for the *CRC Handbook of Toxicology* were reprinted directly from or contain information from numerous previously published sources, I cannot attest to the accuracy and/or completeness of such information and cannot assume any liability of any kind resulting from the use or reliance on the information provided. Mention of vendors, trade names, or commercial products does not constitute endorsement or recommendation for use.

ACKNOWLEDGMENTS

This book would not have been possible without the secretarial skills of Mrs. Rita Levy and the efforts of the following contributors to the *CRC Handbook of Toxicology* from which the tables and figures in this book were reprinted: M.B Abou-Donia, C.S. Auletta, K.L. Bonnette, D.A. Douds, B.J. Dunn, D.J. Ecobichon, H.C. Fogle, R.M. Hoar, M.A. Hollinger, R.V. House, B.S. Levine, K.M. MacKenzie, T.N. Merriman, P.E. Newton, J.C. Peckham, W.J. Powers, R.E. Rush, G.M. Rutledge, G.E. Schulze, J.C. Siglin, and P.T. Thomas.

TABLE OF CONTENTS

Section 1   Laboratory Animals

Section 2   Acute/Chronic Toxicology

Section 3   Dermal Toxicology

Section 4   Ocular Toxicology

Section 5   Inhalation Toxicology

Section 6 Neurotoxicology

Section 7 Immunotoxicology

Section 8 Carcinogenesis

Section 9   Reproductive/Developmental Toxicology

Section 10   Clinical Pathology

Section 11   Risk Assessment

Section 12   Regulatory Toxicology

Section 13   General Information

Section 1:
Laboratory Animals

Table 1 Guiding Principles in the Use of Animals in Toxicology

1. Training and research involving animals should incorporate procedures that are designed and performed with due consideration of current scientific knowledge, the relevance to human or animal health, the advancement of the science of toxicology, and the potential to benefit society.

2. Alternative techniques not involving whole animals should be considered.

3. If alternative techniques cannot be used, the species should be carefully selected and the number of animals kept to the minimum required to achieve reproducible and scientifically valid results.

4. Whenever possible, procedures with animals should avoid or minimize discomfort, distress, and pain.

5. Whenever possible, procedures that may cause more than momentary or slight discomfort, distress, or pain to the animals should be performed with appropriate sedation, analgesia, or anesthesia. Appropriate anesthetics (not muscle relaxants or paralytics) should be used with surgical procedures.

6. The transportation, care, and use of animals should be in accordance with the most current applicable animal welfare acts, federal laws, guidelines, and policies.

7. Care and handling of all animals used for research purposes must be directed by veterinarians or other individuals trained and experienced in the proper care, handling, and use of the species being maintained or studied. When needed, veterinary care shall be provided.

8. Investigators and other personnel shall be appropriately qualified and trained for conducting procedures on living animals. Adequate arrangements shall be made for their training, including training in the proper and humane care and use of laboratory animals.

9. An appropriate review group such as an institutional animal research committee should be responsible for review and approval of protocols involving the use of animals.

10. Euthanasia shall be conducted according to the report of the American Veterinary Medical Association Panel on Euthanasia (*J. Am. Vet. Med. Assoc.*, 1988(3), 252–268, 1986).

From: Society of Toxicology. Guiding Principles in the Use of Animals in Toxicology (adopted 1989). With permission.

Table 2   General Information Sources for the Care and Use of Research Animals

1. *Guide for the Care and Use of Laboratory Animals*, U.S. Department of Health and Human Services, Public Health Service, National Institutes of Health, NIH Publication No. 86–23, Revised 1985 or Succeeding Revised Editions.

2. The Act of August 24, 1986 (Public Law 89-554), commonly known as the Laboratory Welfare Act as amended by the Act of December 24, 1970 (Public Law 91-579), the Animal Welfare Act of 1970, and the Act of April 22, 1976 (Public Law 94-279), the Animal Welfare Act Amendments of 1976, and the Act of December 23, 1985 (Public Law 99-189), (The Food Security Act of 1985) and as it may be subsequently amended; copies may be obtained from the deputy Administrator, U.S. Department of Agriculture, APHIS-VS Federal Building, 6505 Belcrest Road, Hyattsville, MD 20782.

3. Use of Laboratory Animals in Biomedical and Behavioral Research, Committee on the Use of Laboratory Animals in Biomedical and Behavioral Research, Commission on Life Sciences, National Research Council, Institute of Medicine, National Academy Press, Washington, D.C., 1988.

4. International Guiding Principles for Biomedical Research Involving Animals, Council for International Organizations of Medical Sciences (CIOMS), Geneva, 1985.

5. Interdisciplinary Principles and Guidelines for the Use of Animals in Research, Testing and Education, Ad Hoc Animal Research Committee, New York Academy of Sciences, 1988.

Compiled by the Society of Toxicology.

Table 3   Approximate Daily Food and Water Requirements for Various Species

Species	Daily Food Requirement	Daily Water Requirement
Mouse	3–6 g	3–7 ml
Rat	10–20 g	20–30 ml
Hamster	7–15 g	7–15 ml
Guinea pig	20–30 g[a]	12–15 ml/100 g
Rabbit	75–100 g	80–100 ml/kg
Cat	100–225 g	100–200 ml
Dog	250–1200 g	100–400 ml/day
Primate	40 g/kg[a]	350–1000 ml

[a]Like humans, guinea pigs and non-human primates require a continuous supply of vitamin C (ascorbic acid) in the diet.

Table 4 Typical Routes and Dosages of Several Sedative, Analgesic, and Anesthetic Agents

Agents	Dosage and Route in Species						
	Mouse	Rat	Hamster	Guinea Pig	Rabbit	Dog	Primate
Chlorpromazine (mg/kg)	3–35 (IM) 6 (IP)	1–20 (IM) 4–8 (IP)	0.05 (IM)	5–10 (IM)	10–25 (IM)	1–6 (IM) 0.5–8 (PO)	1–6 (IM)
Promazine (mg/kg)	0.5 (IM)	0.5–1 (IM)	0.5–1 (IM)	0.5–1 (IM)	1–2 (IM)	2–4 (IM)	2–4 (IM)
Acepromazine (mg/kg)	—	—	—	—	1 (IM)	0.5–1 (IM) 1–3 (PO)	0.5–1 (IM)
Meperidine (mg/kg)	60 (IM) 40 (IP)	44 (IM) 50 (IP) 25 (IV)	2 (IM)	1 (IP) 2 (IM)	10 (IV)	0.4–10 (IM)	3–11 (IM)
Innovar-Vet (ml/kg)	0.05 (IM)	0.13–0.16 (IM)	—	0.08–0.66 (IM)	0.2–0.3 (IM)	0.13–0.15 (IM)	0.05 (IM)
Ketamine (mg/kg)	25 (IV) 25–50 (IP) 22 (IM)	25 (IV) 50 (IP) 22 (IM)	40 (IM) 100 (IP)	22–64 (IM)	22–44 (IM)	—	5–15 (IM)
Pentobarbital (mg/kg)	35 (IV) 40–70 (IP)	25 (IV) 40–50 (IP)	50–90 (IP)	24 (IV) 30 (IP)	25 (IV) 40 (IP)	30 (IV)	25–35 (IV)
Thiopental (mg/kg)	25–50 (IV)	40 (IM) 25–48 (IP)	—	55 (IM) 20 (IP)	25–50 (IV)	16 (IV)	25 (IV)

Note: Drugs and dosages presented are to serve only as guidelines. Selection and administration of specific agents and dosages should be supervised by a qualified veterinarian. See Chapter 22, Section 9, *CRC Handbook of Toxicology*, Derelanko, M.J. and Hollinger, M.A., Eds., CRC Press, Boca Raton, 1995, for additional information on anesthetics.

Table 5   Summary of the Characteristics of Several Euthanasia Methods

Euthanasia Method	Classification	Mechanism of Action	Species	Effectiveness	Personnel Safety
Inhalant anesthetics	Acceptable	Hypoxia due to depression of vital centers	Small animals such as rats, mice, hamsters, and guinea pigs via chamber administration	Moderately rapid onset of anesthesia; initial excitation may occur	Minimize exposure to personnel by scavenging or venting
Carbon dioxide	Acceptable	Hypoxia due to depression of vital centers	Small animals such as rats, mice, hamsters, and guinea pigs via chamber administration	Effective in adult animals; may be prolonged in immature and neonatal animals	Minimal hazard
Carbon monoxide	Acceptable	Hypoxia due to inhibition of O_2– carry capacity of hemoglobin	Most small species, including dogs, cats, and rodents	Effective and acceptable with proper equipment and operation	Extremely hazardous, difficult to detect
Barbiturates	Acceptable	Hypoxic due to depression of vital centers	Most species	Highly effective when administered appropriately	Safe, except human abuse potential of controlled substance(s)
Inert gases (Ni, Ar)	Conditionally acceptable	Hypoxic hypoxemia	Cats, small dogs, rodents, rabbits, and other small species	Effective, but other methods are preferable; acceptable only if animal is heavily sedated or anesthetized	Safely used in ventilated area

Cervical dislocation	Conditionally acceptable	Hypoxia due to disruption of vital centers, direct depression of brain	Mice, rats <200 g, and rabbits <1 kg	Effective and irreversible; requires training, skill, and IACUC approval; aesthetically displeasing	Safe
Decapitation	Conditionally acceptable	Hypoxia due to disruption of vital centers, direct depression of brain	Rodents and small rabbits	Effective and irreversible; requires training, skill, and IACUC approval; aesthetically displeasing	Potential injury due to guillotine

Table 6   Common Strains of Laboratory Mice

Strain	Description
CD-1 mice	Outbred albino strain descended from "Swiss" mice
CF-1 mice	Outbred albino strain not descended from "Swiss" mice
Swiss-Webster mice	Outbred albino strain from selective inbreeding of Swiss mice by Dr. Leslie Webster
SKH1 (Hairless) mice	Outbred strain that originated from an uncharacterized strain
BALB/c mice	Inbred albino strain developed originally by H.J. Bagg (Bagg albino)
C3H mice	Inbred agouti strain developed originally from "Bagg albino" female and DBA male
C57BL/6 mice	Inbred black strain developed originally by C.C. Little
DBA/2 mice	Inbred non-agouti, dilute brown strain developed originally by C.C. Little; oldest of all inbred mouse strains
FVB mice	Inbred albino strain derived originally from outbred Swiss colony
AKR mice	Inbred albino strain originally developed by Furth as a high leukemia strain
B6C3F1 mice	Hybrid agouti strain from female C57BL/6N × male C3H/He
DBF1 mice	Hybrid black strain from female C57BL/6N × male DBA/2N
CAF1 mice	Hybrid albino strain from female BALB/cAn × male A/HeN
CDF1 mice	Hybrid brown strain from female BALB/cAnN × male DBA/2N
CB6F1 mice	Hybrid black strain from female BALB/cAnN × male C57BL/6N
Nude CD-1 mice	Outbred hairless albino strain that is athymic and thus immunodeficient (unable to produce T-cells)
Nude BALB/cAnN mice	Inbred hairless albino strain that is athymic and thus immunodeficient (unable to produce T-cells)

Table 7   Common Strains of Laboratory Rats

Strain	Description
Sprague-Dawley rats	Outbred albino strain originated by R.W. Dawley from a hybrid hooded male and female Wistar rat
Wistar rats	Outbred albino strain originated at the Wistar Institute
Long-Evans rats	Outbred white with black or occasional brown hood; originated by Drs. Long and Evans by cross of white Wistar females with wild gray male
Zucker rats	Outbred obese strain with four principal coat colors (predominately brown; brown + white; predominately black; or black + white)
Fischer 344 (F-344) rats	Inbred albino strain originated from mating #344 of rats obtained from local breeder (Fischer)
Lewis rats	Inbred albino strain originally developed by Dr. Lewis from Wistar stock
Wistar Kyoto (WKY) rats	Inbred albino strain originated from outbred Wistar stock from Kyoto School of Medicine
Brown Norway rats	Inbred non-agouti brown strain originated from a brown mutation in a stock of rats trapped from the wild at the Wistar Institute in 1930
Spontaneously hypertensive (SHR) rats	Inbred albino strain developed from Wistar Kyoto rats with spontaneous hypertension

Section 2: Acute/Chronic Toxicology

Table 8   Organ Weight Requirements — Standard Study Guidelines

Organ to be Weighed	OECD	JMHW	RDBK	FIFRA[b]	JMAFF	TSCA	MITI
				Guideline[a]			
Adrenal glands	×	×	×		×	×	×
Kidneys	×	×	×	×	×	×	×
Liver	×	×	×	×	×	×	×
Testes	×	×	×	×	×	×	×
Ovaries		×				×	×
Thyroid/ parathyroids	NR	c	NR	NR[d]	NR	NR	
Brain		×		Chronic	Chronic	Chronic	Chronic
Heart		×					Chronic
Lungs		c					Chronic
Spleen		×					Chronic
Pituitary		×					Chronic
Salivary gland		c					
Seminar vesicles		c					
Thymus		c					
Uterus		c					

[a] EC guidelines do not specify organs to be weighed. NR = non-rodent.
[b] Organ weights not required for FIFRA 21- or 90-day dermal studies.
[c] Guidelines state that these organs are "often weighed."
[d] Subchronic studies only.

Table 9   Microscopic Pathology Requirements — Standard Study Guidelines — Tissues Most Often Recommended for Chronic Studies

Tissues[a]	OECD	EC	JMHW	RDBK	FIFRA	JMAFF	TSCA	MITI
Adrenal glands	×	×	×	×	×	×	×	×
Bone (sternum/ femur/ vertebrae)	S, F	S, F or V	S, F	S	S and/or F	S, F	S and/or F	F or V, S
Bone marrow (sternum/ femur/ vertebrae)	S	S, F or V	S, F	S	S and/or F	S, F	S and/or F	S
Brain (medulla/ pons, cerebrum, cerebellum)	×	×	×	×	×	×	×	×
Esophagus	×	×	×	×	×	×	×	×
Heart	×	×	×	×	×	×	×	×
Kidney	×	×	×	×	×	×	×	×
Large intestine (cecum, colon, rectum)	×	Colon	×	×	×	×	×	×
Liver	×	×	×	×	×	×	×	×
Lung (with mainstem bronchi)	×	×	×	×	×	×	×	×
Lymph node (represent- ative)	×	×	×	×	×	×	×	×
Mammary gland	♀[a]	×	×	×	♀	♀	♀	♀
Ovaries	×	×	×	×		×	×	×
Pancreas	×	×	×	×	×	×	×	×
Pituitary	×	×	×	×	×	×	×	×
Prostate	×	×	×	×	×	×	×	×
Salivary glands	×	×	×	×	×	×	×	×
Small intestine (duodenum, ileum, jejunum)	×	×	×	×	×	×	×	×
Spleen	×	×	×	×	×	×	×	×
Stomach	×	×	×	×	×	×	×	×
Testes (with epididymides)	×	×	×	×	×	×	×	×

Table 9   Microscopic Pathology Requirements — Standard Study Guidelines — Tissues Most Often Recommended for Chronic Studies (Continued)

Tissues[a]	OECD	EC	JMHW	RDBK	FIFRA	JMAFF	TSCA	MITI
Thymus	×	×	×	×	×	×	×	×
Thyroid (with parathyroids)	×	×	×	×	×	×	×	×
Trachea	×	×	×	×	×	×	×	×
Urinary bladder	×	×	×	×	×	×	×	×
Uterus	×	×	×	×	×	×	×	×
Gross lesions/ masses/target organs	×	×	×	×	×	×	×	×

[a] ♀ from females.

Table 10 Common Abbreviations and Codes Used in Histopathology

Code	Finding or Observation
+ (1)	= Minimal grade lesion
++ (2)	= Mild or slight grade lesion
+++ (3)	= Moderate grade lesion
++++ (4)	= Marked or severe grade lesion
+++++ (5)	= Very severe or massive grade lesion
(No Entry)	= Lesion not present or organ/tissue not examined
+	= Tissue examined microscopically
–	= Organ/tissue present, no lesion in section
A	= Autolysis precludes examination
B	= Primary benign tumor
I	= Incomplete section of organ/tissue or insufficient tissue for evaluation
M	= Primary malignant tumor
M	= Organ/tissue missing, not present in section
N	= No section of organ/tissue
N	= Normal, organ/tissue within normal limits
NCL	= No corresponding lesion for gross finding
NE	= Organ/tissue not examined
NRL	= No remarkable lesion, organ/tissue within normal limits
NSL	= No significant lesion, organ/tissue within normal limits
P	= Lesion present, not graded (for example, cyst, anomaly)
R	= Recut of section with organ/tissue
U	= Unremarkable organ/tissue, within normal limits
WNL	= Organ/tissues within normal limits
X	= Not remarkable organ/tissue, normal
X	= Incidence of listed morphology, lesion present

Table 11 Frequently Used Grading Schemes for Histopathology

Severity Degree	Proportion of Organ Affected	(A) Grade	Percentage of Organ Affected	(B) Grade	Percentage of Organ Affected	(C) Grade	Percentage of Organ Affected	(D) Grade	Percentage of Organ Affected	(E) Grade	Quantifiable Finding
Minimal	Very small amount	1	(A1) ≤ 1–25% / (A2) < 1–15%	1	<1%	1	<1%	1	<1%	1	
Slight	Very small to small amount			2	1–25%	1	1–25%			1	1–4 foci
Mild	Small amount	2	(A1) 26–50% / (A2) 16–35%			2	26–50%	2	1–30%	2	5–8 foci
Moderate	Middle or median amount	3	(A1) 51–75% / (A2) 36–60%	3	26–50%	3	51–76%	3	31–60%	3	9–12 foci
Marked	Large amount	4	(A1) 76–100% / (A2) 61–100%							4	>12 foci
Moderately severe	Large amount			4	51–75%						
Severe	Very large amount			5	76–100%	4	76–100%	4	81–90%		
Very severe or massive	Very large amount							5	91–100%		

Source: Adapted from Hardisty, J.F. and Eustis, S.L. (1990)[1]; World Health Organization (1978)[2].

Table 12 Suggested Dose Volumes (ml/kg) for Test Material Administration

Species	Gavage		Dermal		IV		IP		SC		IM	
	Ideal	Limit	Ideal	Limit	Ideal	Limit	Ideal	Limit	Ideal	Limit	Ideal	Limit
Mouse	10	20–50	—	—	5	15–25	5–10	30–50	1–5	10–20	0.1	0.5–1
Rat	10	20–50	2	6	1–5	10–20	5–10	10–20	1	10–20	0.1–1	1–10
Rabbit	10	10–20	2	8	1–3	5–10	—	—	1–2.5	5–10	0.1–0.5	1
Dog	10	10–20	—	—	1	5–10	3	5	0.5	1–2	0.1–0.2	1
Monkey	10	10	—	—	1	5–10	3	5	0.5	1–2	0.1–0.5	1

Source: Adapted from *SYNAPSE,* American Society of Laboratory Animal Practitioners (1991).[3] Some adaptations have been made based on experience.

Table 13 Suggested Dosing Apparatus/Needle Sizes (Gauge) for Test Material Administration

Species	Gavage Recommended	Route IV Ideal	IV Range	Ip Ideal	Ip Range	SC Ideal	SC Range	Im Ideal	Im Range
Mouse	Premature infant feeding tube cut to 70 mm, marked at 38 mm	25 or 27	25–30	25 or 27	22–30	25 or 27	22–30	25 or 27	22–30
Rat	3-inch ball-tipped intubation needle	25	25–30	25	22–30	25	25–30	25	22–30
Rabbit	No. 18 French catheter, cut to 15 inches, marked at 12 inches	21	22–30	21	18–23	25	22–25	25	22–30
Dog	Kaslow stomach tube 12Fr ≥ 24 inches; Davol 32Fr intubation tube	21	21–22	—	—	22	20–23	21 or 25	20–25
Monkey	No. 8 French tube (nasogastric gavage)	25	21–22	—	—	22	22–25	25	22–25

Note: Recommended gavage equipment and ideal needle sizes are based on laboratory experience. Suggested ranges of needle sizes are from *Laboratory Manual for Basic Biomethodology of Laboratory Animals*, MTM Associates, Inc.[4]

Table 14   Body Weight: Surface Area Conversion Table

Species	Representative Body Weight to Surface Area[a]		
	Body Weight (kg)	**Surface Area (m^2)**	**Conversion Factor (km)**
Mouse	0.02	0.0066	3
Rat	0.15	0.025	5.9
Monkey	3	0.24	12
Dog	8	0.4	20
Human			
Child	20	0.8	25
Adult	60	1.6	37

[a] Example: To express a mg/kg dose in any given species as the equivalent mg/m^2 dose, multiply the dose by the appropriate km. In human adults, 100 mg/kg is equivalent to 100 mg/kg $\times$ 37 kg/m^2 = 3700 mg/m^2.

Source: Adapted from Freireich, E.J. et al. (1966).[5]

Table 15   Equivalent Surface Area Dosage Conversion Factors

		TO				
		Mouse (20 g)	**Rat (150 g)**	**Monkey (3 kg)**	**Dog (8 kg)**	**Human (60 kg)**
	Mouse	1	1/2	1/4	1/6	1/12
F	Rat	2	1	1/2	1/3	1/6
R	Monkey	4	2	1	3/5	1/3
O	Dog	6	4	3/2	1	1/2
M	Man	12	7	3	2	1

Example: To convert a dose of 50 mg/kg in the mouse to an equivalent dose in the monkey, assuming equivalency on the basis of mg/m^2; multiply 50 mg/kg $\times$ 1/4 = 13 mg/kg.

Note: This table gives approximate factors for converting doses expressed in terms of mg/kg from one species to an equivalent surface area dose expressed as mg/kg in the other species tabulated.

Source: Adapted from Freireich, E.J. et al. (1966).[5]

Table 16 Comparison of Dosage by Weight and Surface Area

Species	Weight (g)	Dosage (mg/kg)	Dose (mg/animal)	Surface Area (cm²)	Dosage (mg/cm²)
Mouse	20	100	2	46	0.043
Rat	200	100	20	325	0.061
Guinea pig	400	100	40	565	0.071
Rabbit	1,500	100	150	1,270	0.110
Cat	2,000	100	200	1,380	0.145
Monkey	4,000	100	400	2,980	0.134
Dog	12,000	100	1,200	5,770	0.207
Human	70,000	100	7,000	18,000	0.388

Source: From Amdur, M.O., Doull, J., and Klaassen, C.D., Eds. (1991).[6] With permission.

Table 17 Approximate Diet Conversion Factors (ppm to mg/kg)

Species	Age	Conversion Factor (divide ppm by)
Mice	Young (1–12 wk of study)	5
	Older (13–78 wk of study)	6–7
Rats	Young (1–12 wk of study)	10
	Older (13–104 wk of study)	20
Dogs		40

Note: To estimate the approximate test material of rats receiving a 1000-ppm dietary concentration during a 4-week study: 1000 ppm ÷ 10 = 100 mg/kg b.w./day.

Table 18 Clinical Signs of Toxicity

	Clinical Observation		Observed Signs	Organs, Tissues, of Systems Most Likely to be Involved
I.	Respiratory: blockage in the nostrils, changes in rate and depth of breathing, changes in color of body surfaces	A.	Dyspnea: difficult or labored breathing, essentially gasping for air, respiration rate usually slow	
			1. Abdominal breathing: breathing by diaphragm, greater deflection of abdomen upon inspiration	CNS respiratory center, paralysis of costal muscles, cholinergic inhibition
			2. Gasping: deep labored inspiration, accompanied by a wheezing sound	CNS respiratory center, pulmonary edema, secretion accumulation in airways (increase cholinergic)
		B.	Apnea: a transient cessation of breathing following a forced respiration	CNS respiratory center, pulmonary cardiac insufficiency
		C.	Cyanosis: bluish appearance of tail, mouth, foot pads	Pulmonary-cardiac insufficiency, pulmonary edema
		D.	Tachypnea: quick and usually shallow respiration	Stimulation of respiratory center, pulmonary-cardiac insufficiency
		E.	Nostril discharges: red or colorless	Pulmonary edema, hemorrhage
II.	Motor activities: changes in frequency and nature of movements	A.	Decrease or increase in spontaneous motor activities, curiosity, preening, or locomotions	Somatomotor, CNS
		B.	Somnolence: animal appears drowsy, but can be aroused by prodding and resumes normal activities	CNS sleep center
		C.	Loss of righting reflex: loss of reflex to maintain normal upright posture when placed on the back	CNS, sensory, neuromuscular

Table 18   Clinical Signs of Toxicity (Continued)

Clinical Observation		Observed Signs	Organs, Tissues, of Systems Most Likely to be Involved
	D.	Anesthesia: loss of righting reflex and pain response (animal will not respond to tail and toe pinch)	CNS, sensory
	E.	Catalepsy: animal tends to remain in any position in which it is placed	CNS, sensory, neuromuscular, autonomic
	F.	Ataxia: inability to control and coordinate movement while animal is walking with no spasticity, epraxia, paresis, or rigidity	CNS, sensory, autonomic
	G.	Unusual locomotion: spastic, toe walking, pedaling, hopping, and low body posture	CNS, sensory, neuromuscular
	H.	Prostration: immobile and rests on belly	CNS, sensory, neuromuscular
	I.	Tremors: involving trembling and quivering of the limbs or entire body	Neuromuscular, CNS
	J.	Fasciculation: involving movements of muscles, seen on the back, shoulders, hind limbs, and digits of the paws	Neuromuscular, CNS, autonomic
III. Convulsion (seizure): marked involuntary contraction or seizures of contraction of voluntary muscle	A.	Clonic convulsion: convulsive alternating contraction and relaxation of muscles	CNS, respiratory failure, neuromuscular, autonomic
	B.	Tonic convulsion: persistent contraction of muscles, attended by rigid extension of hind limbs	
	C.	Tonic-clonic convulsion: both types may appear consecutively	

Table 18   Clinical Signs of Toxicity (Continued)

Clinical Observation		Observed Signs	Organs, Tissues, of Systems Most Likely to be Involved
	D.	Asphyxial convulsion: usually of clonic type, but accompanied by gasping and cyanosis	
	E.	Opisthotonos: tetanic spasm in which the back is arched and the head is pulled toward the dorsal position	
IV. Reflexes	A.	Corneal (eyelid closure): touching of the cornea causes eyelids to close	Sensory, neuromuscular
	B.	Pinnal: twitch of external ear elicited by light stroking of inside surface of ear	Sensory, neuromuscular, autonomic
	C.	Righting	CNS, sensory, neuromuscular
	D.	Myotact: ability of animal to retract its hind limb when limb is pulled down over the edge of a surface	Sensory, neuromuscular
	E.	Light (pupillary): constriction of pupil in the presence of light	Sensory, neuromuscular, autonomic
	F.	Startle reflex: response to external stimuli such as touch, noise	Sensory, neuromuscular
V. Ocular signs	A.	Lacrimation: excessive tearing, clear or colored	Autonomic
	B.	Miosis: constriction of pupil regardless of the presence or absence of light	Autonomic
	C.	Mydriasis: dilation of pupils regardless of the presence or absence of light	Autonomic
	D.	Exophthalmos: abnormal protrusion of eye from orbit	Autonomic
	E.	Ptosis: dropping of upper eyelids, not reversed by prodding animal	Autonomic

Table 18 Clinical Signs of Toxicity (Continued)

	Clinical Observation		Observed Signs	Organs, Tissues, of Systems Most Likely to be Involved
		F.	Chromodacryorrhea (red lacrimation)	Autonomic, hemorrhage, infection
		G.	Relaxation of nictitating membrane	Autonomic
		II.	Corneal opacity, iritis, conjunctivitis	Irritation of the eye
VI.	Cardiovascular signs	A.	Bradycardia: decreased heart rate	Autonomic, pulmonary-cardiac insufficiency
		B.	Tachycardia: increased heart rate	Autonomic, pulmonary-cardiac insufficiency
		C.	Vasodilation: redness of skin, tall, tongue, ear, foot pad, conjunctivae, and warm body	Autonomic, CNS, increased cardiac output, hot environment
		D.	Vasoconstriction: blanching or whitening of skin, cold body	Autonomic, CNS, cold environment, cardiac output decrease
		E.	Arrhythmia: abnormal cardiac rhythm	CNS, autonomic, cardiac-pulmonary insufficiency, myocardial infarction
VII.	Salivation	A.	Excessive secretion of saliva: hair around mouth becomes wet	Autonomic
VIII.	Piloerection	A.	Contraction of erectile tissue of hair follicles resulting in rough hair	Autonomic
IX.	Analgesia	A.	Decrease in reaction to induced pain (e.g., hot plate)	Sensory, CNS
X.	Muscle tone	A.	Hypotonia: generalized decrease in muscle tone	Autonomic
		B.	Hypertonia: generalized increase in muscle tension	Autonomic

Table 18   Clinical Signs of Toxicity (Continued)

	Clinical Observation		Observed Signs	Organs, Tissues, of Systems Most Likely to be Involved
XI.	Gastrointestinal signs: dropping (feces)	A.	Solid, dried, and scant	Autonomic, constipation, GI motility
		B.	Loss of fluid, watery stool	Autonomic, diarrhea, GI motility
	Emesis	A.	Vomiting and retching	Sensory, CNS, autonomic (in rat, emesis is absent)
	Diuresis	A.	Red urine (hematuria)	Damage in kidney
		B.	Involuntary urination	Autonomic, sensory
XII.	Skin	A.	Edema: swelling of tissue filled with fluid	Irritation, renal failure, tissue damage, long-term immobility
		B.	Erythema: redness of skin	Irritation, inflammation, sensitization

Source: From Chan, P.K. and Hayes, A.W. (1989).[7] With permission.

Table 19   Autonomic Signs

Sympathomimetic	Piloerection
	Partial mydriasis
Sympathetic block	Ptosis
	Diagnostic if associated with sedation
Parasympathomimetic	Salivation (examined by holding blotting paper)
	Miosis
	Diarrhea
	Chromodacryorrhea in rats
Parasympathomimetic block	Mydriasis (maximal)
	Excessive dryness of mouth (detect with blotting paper)

Source: From Chan, P.K. and Hayes, A.W. (1989).[7] With permission.

Table 20   Toxic Signs of Acetylcholinesterase Inhibition

Muscarinic Effects[a]	Nicotinic Effects[b]	CNS Effects[c]
Bronchoconstriction	Muscular twitching	Giddiness
Increased bronchosecretion	Fasciculation	Anxiety
Nausea and vomiting (absent in rats)	Cramping Muscular weakness	Insomnia Nightmares
Diarrhea		Headache
Bradycardia		Apathy
Hypotension		Depression
Miosis		Drowsiness
Urinary incontinence		Confusion
		Ataxia
		Coma
		Depressed reflex
		Seizure
		Respiratory depression

[a] Blocked by atropine.

[b] Not blocked by atropine

[c] Atropine might block early signs.

Source: From Chan, P.K. and Hayes, A.W. (1989).[7] With permission.

Table 21   Effect of Decreased Body Weights on Relative Organ Weights of Rats

Decrease	No Change	Increase
Liver (?)	Heart	Adrenal glands (?)
	Kidneys	Brain
	Prostate	Epididymides
	Spleen	Pituitary
	Ovaries	Testes
		Thyroid (?)
		Uterus

Note 1: (?) = Differences slight or inconsistent.

Note 2: Relative weights = organ/body weight ratios.

Note 3: For absolute weights, all except thyroids decrease. Summary of results reported in: Schwartz, E., Tomaben, J.A., and Boxill, G.C. (1973)[8]; and Scharer, K. (1977).[9]

References

1. Hardisty, J.F. and Eustis, S.L., Toxicological pathology: a critical stage in study interpretation, in *Progress in Predictive Toxicology*, Clayson, D.B., Munro, I.C., Shubik, P., and Swenberg, J.A., Eds., Elsevier, New York, 1990.

2. World Health Organization, *Principles and Methods for Evaluating the Toxicity of Chemicals. Part I*, Environmental Health Criteria 6, World Health Organization, Geneva, 1978.

3. *SYNAPSE*, American Society of Laboratory Animal Practitioners, Vol. 24, March 1991.

4. *Laboratory Manual for Basic Biomethodology of Laboratory Animals*, MTM Associates, Inc.

5. Freireich, E.J. et al., Quantitative comparison of toxicity of anti-cancer agents in mouse, rat, dog and monkey and man, *Cancer Chemother. Rep.*, 50, 219, 1966.

6. Amdur, M.O., Doull, J., and Klaassen, C.D., Eds., *Casarett and Doull's Toxicology*, 4th ed., Pergamon Press, New York, 1991.

7. Chan, P.K. and Hayes, A.W., Principles and methods for acute toxicity and eye irritancy, in *Principles and Methods of Toxicology*, 2nd ed., A.W. Hayes, Ed., Raven Press, New York, 1989.

8. Schwartz, E., Tomaben, J.A., and Boxill, G.C., The effects of food restriction on hematology, clinical chemistry and pathology in the albino rat, *Toxicol. Appl. Pharmacol.*, 25, 515, 1973.

9. Scharer, K., The effect of underfeeding on organ weights of rats. How to interpret organ weight changes in cases of marked growth retardation in toxicity tests, *Toxicology*, 7, 45, 1977.

Section 3: Dermal Toxicology

Table 22　Draize Dermal Irritation Scoring System

Erythema and Eschar Formation	Value	Edema Formation	Value
No erythema	0	No edema	0
Very slight erythema (barely perceptible)	1	Very slight edema (barely perceptible)	1
Well-defined erythema	2	Slight edema (edges of area well defined by definite raising)	2
Moderate to severe erythema	3	Moderate edema (raised approximately 1 mm)	3
Severe erythema (beet-redness) to slight, eschar formation (injuries in depth)	4	Severe edema (raised more than 1 mm and extending beyond the area of exposure)	4

Source: From Draize, J.H. (1959).[1]

Table 23 Human Patch Test Dermal Irritation Scoring System

Skin Reaction	Value
No sign of inflammation; normal skin	0
Glazed appearance of the sites, or barely perceptible erythema	±(0.5)
Slight erythema	1
Moderate erythema, possible with barely perceptible edema at the margin, papules may be present	2
Moderate erythema, with generalized edema	3
Severe erythema with severe edema, with or without vesicles	4
Severe reaction spread beyond the area of the patch	5

Source: From Patrick E. and Maibach, H.I. (1989).[2]

Table 24 Chamber Scarification Dermal Irritation Scoring System

Skin Reaction	Value
Scratch marks barely visible	0
Erythema confined to scratches perceptible erythema	1
Broader bands of increased erythema, with or without rows of vesicles, pustules, or erosions	2
Severe erythema with partial confluency, with or without other lesions	3
Confluent, severe erythema sometimes associated with edema, necrosis, or bullae	4

Source: From Patrick E. and Maibach, H.I. (1989).[2]

Table 25 Magnusson Sensitization Scoring System

Skin Reaction	Value
No reaction	0
Scattered reaction	1
Moderate and diffuse reaction	2
Intense reddening and swelling	3

Source: From Magnusson, R. and Kligman, A. (1970).[3]

Table 26 Split Adjuvant Sensitization Scoring System

Skin Reaction	Value
Normal skin	0
Very faint, nonconfluent pink	±
Faint pink	+
Pale pink to pink, slight edema	++
Pink, moderate edema	+++
Pink and thickened	++++
Bright pink, markedly thickened	+++++

Source: From Klecak, G. (1983).[4]

Table 27 Buehler Sensitization Scoring System

Skin Reaction	Value
No reaction	0
Very faint erythema, usually confluent	±(0.5)
Faint erythema, usually confluent	1
Moderate erythema	2
Strong erythema, with or without edema	3

Source: From Buehler, E.V. and Griffin, F. (1975).[5]

Table 28 Contact Photosensitization Scoring System

Skin Reaction	Value
No erythema	0
Minimal but definite erythema confluent	1
Moderate erythema	2
Considerable erythema	3
Maximal erythema	4

Source: From Harber, L.C., Shalita, A.R., and Armstrong, R.B. (1993).[6]

Table 29 Human Patch Test Sensitization Scoring System

Skin Reaction	Value
Doubtful reaction; faint erythema only	? or + ?
Weak positive reaction; erythema, infiltration, discrete papules	+
Strong positive reaction; erythema, infiltration, papules, vesicles	++
Extreme positive reaction, intense erythema, infiltration, and coalescing vesicles	+++
Negative reaction	–
Irritant reaction of different types	IR
Not tested	NT

Source: From Fischer, T. and Maibach, H.I. (1991).[7]

Table 30 Environmental Protection Agency (EPA) Method of Calculating the Primary Irritation Index (PII) for Dermal Irritation Studies

Option 1

Separately add up each animal's erythema and edema scores for the 1-, 24-, 48-, and 72-hr scoring intervals. Add all six values together and divide by the (number of test sites × 4 scoring intervals).

Option 2

Add the 1-, 24-, 48-, and 72-hr erythema and edema scores for all animals and divide by the (number of test sites × 4 scoring intervals).

Source: From U.S. EPA (1984)[8] and (1992).[9]

Table 31 Federal Hazardous Substances Act (CPSC-FHSA) Method of Calculating the Primary Irritation Index (PII) for Dermal Irritation Studies

Option 1

Separately add up each animal's intact and abraded erythema and edema scores for the 25- and 72-hr scoring intervals. Add all six values together and divide by the (number of test sites × 2 scoring intervals).

Option 2

Add the 25- and 72-hr erythema and edema scores for all animals (intact and abraded sites) and divide by the (number of test sites × 2 scoring intervals).

Source: From U.S. Consumer Products Safety Commission (1993).[10]

Table 32 European Economic Community's (EEC) Method of Calculating the Primary Irritation Index (PII) for Dermal Irritation Studies

1. *Erythema*: Add all 24-, 48-, and 72-hr erythema scores for each animal together and divide by the (number of test sites × 3 scoring intervals).

2. *Edema*: Add all 24-, 48-, and 72-hr edema scores for each animal together and divide by the (number of test sites × 3 scoring intervals).

Source: From the Commission of the European Communities (1992).[11]

Table 33   Environmental Protection Agency (EPA) Dermal Classification System

Primary Irritation Index	Irritation Rating
0.00	Nonirritant
0.01–1.99	Slight irritant
2.00–5.00	Moderate irritant
5.01–8.00	Severe irritant

Source: From U.S. EPA (1988).[12]

Table 34   Environmental Protection Agency (EPA) Standard Evaluation Procedure Dermal Classification System

Mean Score (Primary Irritation Index)	Response Category
0–0.4	Negligible
0.5–1.9	Slight
2–4.9	Moderate
5–8.0	Strong (primary irritant)

Source: From U.S. EPA (1984).[13]

Table 35   Federal Fungicide, Insecticide, and Rodenticide Act (EPA-FIFRA) Dermal Classification System

Toxicity Category	Warning Label
I	Corrosive. Causes eye and skin damage (or irritation). Do not get in eyes, on skin, or on clothing. Wear goggles or face shield and gloves when handling. Harmful or fatal if swallowed. (Appropriate first aid statement required.)
II	Severe irritation at 72 hr. Causes eye (and skin) irritation. Do not get on skin or on clothing. Harmful if swallowed. (Appropriate first aid statement required.)
III	Moderate irritation at 72 hr. Avoid contact with skin, eyes, or clothing. In case of contact, immediately flush eyes or skin with plenty of water. Get medical attention if irritation persists.
IV	Mild or slight irritation at 72 hr. (No precautionary statements required.)

Source: From U.S. EPA (1993).[14]

Table 36   European Economic Community (EEC) Dermal Classification System

Mean Erythema Score	Irritation Rating
0.00–1.99	Nonirritant
≥ 2.00	Irritant

Mean Edema Score	Irritation Rating
0.00–1.99	Nonirritant
≥ 2.00	Irritant

Source: From the Commission of the European Communities (1983).[15]

Table 37   Federal Hazardous Substances Act (CPSC-FHSA) Dermal Classification System

Primary Irritation Score	Irritation Rating
0.00–4.99	Nonirritant
≥5.00	Irritant

Source: From U.S. Consumer Products Safety Commission (1993).[10]

Table 38   Draize Dermal Classification System

Primary Irritation Index	Irritation Rating
<2	Mildly irritating
2–5	Moderately irritating
>5	Severely irritating

Source: From Patrick E. and Maibach, H.I. (1989).[2]

Table 39   Department of Transportation (DOT) and International Maritime Organization (IMO) Packing Group Classification System

Packing Group	Definition
I[a]	Substances that cause visible destruction or irreversible alterations of the skin tissue at the site of contact when tested on the intact skin of an animal for not more than 3 min.
II	Substances that cause visible destruction or irreversible alterations of the skin tissue at the site of contact when tested on the intact skin or an animal for not more than 60 min.
III	Substances that cause visible destruction or irreversible alterations of the skin tissue at the site of contact when tested on the intact skin of an animal for not more than 4 hr or which have a corrosion rate on steel or aluminum surfaces exceeding 6.25 mm (0.246 inches) a year at a test temperature of 55°C (131°F).

[a] Current DOT regulations (1998) indicate effects should occur within 60 minutes of exposure in order to be assigned to Packing Group I.

Source: From International Maritime Dangerous Goods Code (1994)[16]; U.S. Occupational Safety and Health Administration (1991).[17]

Table 40   Maximization Sensitization Classification System

Sensitization Rate, %	Grade	Classification
0	—	Nonsensitizer
>0–8	I	Weak sensitizer
9–28	II	Mild sensitizer
29–64	III	Moderate sensitizer
65–80	IV	Strong sensitizer
81–100	V	Extreme sensitizer

Source: From Magnusson, B. and Kligman, A. (1970).[3]

Table 41   Optimization Sensitization Classification System

Intradermal Positive Animals %	Epidermal Positive Animals %	Classification
s, >75	and/or s, >50	Strong sensitizer
s, 50–75	and/or s, 30–50	Moderate sensitizer
s, 30–50	n.s., 0–30	Weak sensitizer
n.s., 0–30	n.s., 0	No sensitizer

Note: s, significant; n.s., not significant (using Fisher's Exact Test).

Source: From Patrick, E. and Maibach, H.I. (1989).[2]

Table 42 Common Materials Used as Positive Controls

Material	CAS No.	Suggested Concentrations	Category
Sodium lauryl sulfate	151-21-3	1.0%	Irritant
Hexyl cinnamic aldehyde	101-86-0	—	Mild to moderate sensitizer
Mercaptobenzothiazole	149-30-4	—	Mild to moderate sensitizer
Benzocaine	94-09-7	—	Mild to moderate sensitizer
p-Phenylenediamine	106-50-3	—	Sensitizer
2,4-Dinitrochlorobenzene (DNCB)	97-00-7	Induction: 0.1% to 0.5%, 0.25% w/v in ethanol/acetone Challenge: 0.1 to 0.3%, w/v in ethanol/acetone	Sensitizer
Potassium dichromate	7778-50-9	—	Sensitizer
Neomycin sulfate	1405-10-3	—	Sensitizer
Nickel sulfate	7786-81-4	—	Sensitizer
8-Methoxypsoralen (Oxsoralen Lotion®)	298-81-7	1.0%	Photoirritant
5-Methoxypsoralen (Bergapten)	298-81-7	1.0%	Photoirritant
2,4-Dinitro-3-methyl-6-tertiary-butylanisole (musk ambrette)	83-66-9	Induction: 10.0% w/v in ethanol/acetone Challenge: 0.5% w/v in ethanol/acetone	Photosensitizer
2-Chloro-10-[3-dimethyl-aminopropyl] pheno-thiazine hydrochloride (chlorpromazine)	50-53-3	Induction: 1.0% w/v in methanol Challenge: 0.1% w/v in methanol	Photosensitizer
3,3,4,5-Tetrachlorosalicylanide (TCSA)	1154-59-2	Induction: 1.0% w/v in acetone Challenge: 1.0% w/v in acetone	Photosensitizer (in mice and guinea pigs), possible sensitizer in guinea pigs

Source: From Organization for Economic Cooperation and Development (1992)[18]; The Commission of the European Communities (1992)[19]; Springborn Laboratories, Inc. (1994)[20]; Hakim, R.E., Freeman, R.G., Griffin, A.C., and Knox, J.M. (1961)[21]; Springborn Laboratories, Inc. (1994)[22]; Siglin, J.C., Jenkins, P.K., Smith, P.S., Ryan, C.A., and Gerberick, G.F. (1991)[23]; Springborn Laboratories, Inc. (1994)[24]; Ichikawa, H., Armstrong, R.B., and Harber, L.C. (1981)[25]; and Springborn Laboratories, Inc. (1994).[26]

References

1. Draize, J.H., *Appraisal of the Safety of Chemicals in Foods, Drugs and Cosmetics*, The Association of Food and Drug Officials of the United States, 49, 1959.

2. Patrick, E. and Maibach, H.I., Dermatotoxicology, in *Principles and Methods of Toxicology*, 2nd edition, Hayes, A.W., Ed., Raven Press, New York, 1989, chap. 32.

3. Magnusson, B. and Kligman, A., *Allergic Contact Dermatitis in the Guinea Pigs*, Charles C Thomas, Springfield, IL, 1970.

4. Klecak, G., Identification of contact allergies: predictive tests in animals, in *Dermatotoxicology*, 2nd edition, Marzulli, F.N. and Maibach, H.I., Eds., Hemisphere Publishing, Washington, D.C., 1983, chap. 9.

5. Buehler, E.V. and Griffin, F., Experimental skin sensitization in the guinea pig and man, *Animal Models Dermatol.*, 55, 1975.

6. Harber, L.C., Shalita, A.R., and Armstrong, R.B., Immunologically mediated contact photosensitivity in guinea pigs, in *Dermatotoxicology*, 2nd edition, Marzulli, F.N. and Maibach, H.I., Eds., Hemisphere Publishing, Washington, D.C., 1993, chap. 16.

7. Fischer, T. and Maibach, H.I., Patch testing in allergic contact dermatitis, in *Exogenous Dermatoses: Environmental Dermatitis*, Menne, T. and Maibach, H.I., Eds., CRC Press, Boca Raton, FL, 1991, chap. 7.

8. United States Environmental Protection Agency, Federal Insecticide, Fungicide, Rodenticide Act, Pesticide Assessment Guidelines, Subdivision F, Hazard Evaluation: Human and Domestic Animals, Series 81-5 Dermal Irritation, 55e, 1984.

9. United States Environmental Protection Agency, Toxic Substances Control Act, Test Guidelines, 40 CFR Part 798, Subpart E — Specific Organ/Tissue Toxicity, Section 798.4470 Primary Dermal Irritation, 491, 1992.

10. United States Consumer Products Safety Commission, 16 CFR Chapter II, Subchapter C: Federal Hazardous Substances Act Regulation, Part 1500, Subsection 1500.3: Definitions, 381, 1993.

11. The Commission of the European Communities, *Official Journal of the European Communities, Part B: Methods for the Determination of Toxicity*, No. L 383 A/124, B.4. Acute Toxicity (Skin Irritation), 1992.

12. United Stated Environmental Protection Agency, Federal Insecticide, Fungicide, Rodenticide Act, Pesticide Assessment Guidelines, Subdivision F: Hazard Evaluation: Humans and Domestic Animals — Addendum 3 on Data Reporting, 1988.

13. United States Environmental Protection Agency, Federal Insecticide, Fungicide, Rodenticide Act, Pesticide Assessment Guidelines, Hazard Evaluation Division, Standard Evaluation Procedure, Guidance for Evaluation of Dermal Irritation Testing, 1, 1984.

14. United States Environmental Protection Agency, Toxic Substances Control Act, Test Guidelines, 40 CFR chap.1 (7-1-93), Part 156: Labeling Requirements for Pesticides and Devices, Section 156.10, 75, 1993.

15. The Commission of the European Communities, *Official Journal of the European Communities, Annex VI, General Classification and Labeling Requirements for Dangerous Substances*, No. L257/11, 1983.

16. International Maritime Dangerous Goods Code, Class 8 Corrosives. International Maritime Organization, London, England, 1994.

17. United States Occupational Safety and Health Administration, Labor, 29 CFR Chapter XVII, Part 1910, Appendix A to Section 1900.1200 — Health Hazard Definitions (Mandatory), 364, 1991.

18. Organization for Economic Cooperation and Development, OECD Guidelines for Testing of Chemicals, Section 4: Health Effects, Subsection 406: Skin Sensitization, 1, 1992.

19. The Commission of the European Communities, *Official Journal of the European Communities, Part B. Methods for the Determination of Toxicity*, No. L 383 A/131, B.6: Skin Sensitization, 1992.

20. Springborn Laboratories, Inc., Protocol for a Primary Irritation Study in Rabbits, EPA/PSI-1 – 2/94, Spencerville, OH, 1994.

21. Hakim, R.E., Freeman, R.G., Griffin, A.C., and Knox, J.M., Experimental toxicologic studies on 8-methoxypsoralen in animals exposed to the long ultraviolet, *J. Pharmacol. Exp. Ther.*, 131, 394, 1961.

22. Springborn Laboratories, Inc., *Protocol for a Photoirritation Study in Rabbits*, FDA/PHI-1-2/94, Spencerville, OH, 1994.

23. Siglin, J.C., Jenkins, P.K., Smith, P.S., Ryan, C.A., and Gerberick, G.F., Evaluation of a New Murine Model for the Predictive Assessment of Contact Photoallergy (CPA), *American College of Toxicology Annual Meeting*, Savannah, GA, 1991.

24. Springborn Laboratories, Inc., *Protocol for a Photoallergy Study in Mice*, FDA/PHS-2-2/94, Spencerville, OH, 1994.

25. Ichikawa, H., Armstrong, R.B., and Harber, L.C., Photoallergic contact dermatitis in guinea pigs; Improved induction technique using Freund's complete adjuvant. *J. Invest. Dermatol.*, 76, 498, 1981.

26. Springborn Laboratories, Inc., *Protocol for a Photosensitization Study in Guinea Pigs*, FDA/PHS-1-2/94, Spencerville, OH, 1994.

Section 4:
Ocular Toxicology

Table 43   Scale of Weighted Scores for Grading the Severity of Ocular Lesions Developed by Draize et al.

In 1994, Draize et al.[1] described an eye irritancy grading system for evaluating drugs and other materials intended for use in or around the eye. Numerical scores were assigned for reactions of cornea, iris, and conjunctiva. The total ocular irritation score was calculated by a formula that gave the greatest weight to corneal changes (total maximum = 80). A total maximum score = 10 for the iris, and 20 for the conjunctiva.

I.   Cornea

    A.   Opacity-Degree of Density (area which is most dense is taken for reading)

        Scattered or diffuse area — details of iris clearly visible....................................1

        Easily discernible translucent areas, details of iris clearly visible......................2

        Opalescent areas, no details of iris visible, size of pupil barely discernible.....3

        Opaque, iris invisible..4

    B.   Area of Cornea Involved

        One quarter (or less) but not zero..1

        Greater than one quarter — less than one half...2

        Greater than one half — less than three quarters..3

        Greater than three quarters — up to whole area..4

        Score equals A × B × 5   Total Maximum = 80

II.   Iris

    A.   Values

        Folds have normal, congestion, swelling, circumcorneal injection
           (any one or all of these or combination of any thereof), iris still reacting
           to light (sluggish reaction is positive)...1

        No reaction to light, hemorrhage; gross destruction (any one or all of these).....2

        Score equals A × 5   Total possible maximum = 10

Table 43   Scale of Weighted Scores for Grading the Severity of Ocular Lesions Developed by Draize et al. (Continued)

III.   Conjunctivae

    A.   Redness (refers to palpebral conjunctivae only)

        Vessels definitely injected above normal..1

        More diffuse, deeper crimson red, individual vessels not easily discernible.....2

        Diffuse beefy red..3

    B.   Chemosis

        Any swelling above normal (includes nictitating membrane)............................1

        Obvious swelling with partial eversion of the lids..2

        Swelling with lids about half closed..3

        Swelling with lids about half closed to completely closed...............................4

    C.   Discharge

        Any amount different from normal (does not include small amounts
          observed in inner canthus of normal animals..1

        Discharge with moistening of the lids and hairs just adjacent to the lids.........2

        Discharge with moistening of the lids and considerable area around the eye.....3

        Score (A + B + C) × 2   Total maximum = 20

Note: The maximum total score is the sum of all scores obtained for the cornea, iris, and conjunctiva.

Table 44   Grades for Ocular Lesions

The following standardized grading system is used in testing guidelines of several U.S. federal agencies (Consumer Product Safety Commission, Occupational Safety and Health Administration, Food and Drug Administration, Environmental Protection Agency, and Food Safety and Quality Service of the Department of Agriculture) and the Organization for Economic Cooperation and Development (OECD) member countries.

Cornea

Opacity: degree of density (area most dense taken for reading)

No ulceration or opacity...0

Scattered or diffuse areas of opacity (other than slight dulling of normal luster, details of iris clearly visible)..1[a]

Easily discernible translucent areas, details of iris slightly obscured............................2

Nacreous areas, no details of iris visible, size of pupil barely discernible.................3

Opaque cornea, iris not discernible through the opacity...4

Iris

Normal... 0

Markedly deepened rugae, congestion, swelling, moderate circumcorneal hyperemia, or injection, any of these or any combination thereof, iris still reacting to light (sluggish reaction is positive... 1[a]

No reaction to light, hemorrhage, gross destruction (any or all of these)....................2

Conjunctivae

Redness (refers to palpebral and bulbar conjunctivae, excluding cornea and iris)

Blood vessels normal..0

Some blood vessels definitely hyperemic (injected)..1

Diffuse, crimson color, individual vessels not easily discernible..................................2[a]

Diffuse beefy red...3

Chemosis: lids and/or nictitating membranes

No swelling...0

Any swelling above normal (includes nictitating membranes)....................................1

Obvious swelling with partial eversion of lids... 2[a]

Swelling with lids about half closed...3

Swelling with lids more than half closed..4

[a]   Readings at these numerical values or greater indicate positive responses.

Table 45   Classification of Compounds Based on Eye Irritation Properties

This classification scheme, developed by Kay and Calandra,[2] utilizes the Draize scoring system to rate the irritating potential of substances.

1.   **Step 1**

Using the Draize eye irritation scoring system, find the maximum mean total score for all three tissues (cornea, iris, and conjunctivae) occurring within the first 96 hours after instillation for which the incidence of this score plus or minus 5 points is at least 40%.

2.   **Step 2**

Choose an initial or "tentative rating" on the basis of the score found in Step 1 as follows:

Score from Step 1	Tentative Eye Irritation Rating	Symbol
0.0–0.5 points	Nonirritating	N
0.5–2.5 points	Practically nonirritating	PN
2.5–15 points	Minimally irritating	M_1
15–25 points	Mildly irritating	M_2
25–50 points	Moderately irritating	M_3
50–80 points	Severely irritating	S
80–100 points	Extremely irritating	E
100–110 points	Maximally irritating	M_x

For borderline scores, choose the higher rating.

3.   **Step 3**

Tentative Rating	Requirement for Maintenance
N	$MTS_{24} = 0$; for $MTS_{24} > 0$, raise one level
PN	As for N
M_1	$MTS_{48} = 0$; for $MTS_{48} > 0$, raise one level
M_2	$MTS_{96} = 0$; for $MTS_{96} > 0$, raise one level
M_3	1. $MTS_f \leq 20$; for $MTS_f > 20$, raise one level
	2. $ITS_f \leq 10$ (60%); if not true, then no rabbit may show ITS_f 30; otherwise, raise one level
S	1. As for M_3 except use $MTS_f \leq 40$
	2. As for M_3 except use $ITS_f \leq 30$ (60%) and 60 for high

Table 45 Classification of Compounds Based on Eye Irritation Properties (Continued)

Tentative Rating	Requirement for Maintenance
E	1. As for M_3 except use $MTS_f \leq 80$
	2. As for M_3 except use $ITS_f \leq 60$ (60%) and 100 for high
M_x	1. $MTS_f > 80$ (60%); for $MTS_f \leq 80$, lower one level
	2. $ITS_f > 60$ (60%); otherwise lower one level

Note 1: Symbols: MTS = mean total score; ITS = individual rabbit total score. Subscripts denote scoring interval: 24, 48, or 96 hr; f = final score (7 days).

Note 2: Two requirements must be met before a tentative rating may become final. First, the mean total score for the 7 day scoring interval may not exceed 20 points if the rating is to be maintained. Second, individual total scores for at least 60% of the rabbits should be 10 points or less and in no case may any individual rabbit's total score exceed 30. If either or both of these requirements are not met, then the "tentative rating" must be raised one level and the higher level becomes the "final rating."

Table 46   NAS Classification Method Based on Severity and Persistence

This descriptive scale, adapted from work conducted by Green et al.,[3] attaches significance to the persistence and reversibility of responses. It is based on the most severe response observed in a group of animals rather than the average response.

1. **Inconsequential or Complete Lack of Irritation**

    Exposure of the eye to a material under the specified conditions causes no significant ocular changes. No staining with fluorescein can be observed. Any changes that occur clear within 24 hours and are no greater than those caused by isotonic saline under the same conditions.

2. **Moderate Irritation**

    Exposure of the eye to the material under the specified conditions causes minor, superficial, and transient changes of the cornea, iris, or conjunctiva as determined by external or slit lamp examination with fluorescein staining. The appearance at the 24-hour or subsequent grading of any of the following changes is sufficient to characterize a response as moderate irritation: opacity of the cornea (other than a slight dulling of the normal luster), hyperemia of the iris, or swelling of the conjunctiva. Any changes that are seen clear up within 7 days.

3. **Substantial Irritation**

    Exposure of the eye to the material under the specified conditions causes significant injury to the eye, such as loss of the corneal epithelium, corneal opacity, iritis (other than a slight injection), conjunctivitis, pannus, or bullae. The effects clear up within 21 days.

4. **Severe Irritation or Corrosion**

    Exposure of the eye to the material under the specified conditions results in the same types of injury as in the previous category and in significant necrosis or other injuries that adversely affect the visual process. Injuries persist for 21 days or more.

Source: From National Academy of Sciences (1977).[4]

Table 47 Modified NAS Classification Method Developed by Brendan J. Dunn, Department of Toxicology and Risk Assessment, Honeywell International Inc. (unpublished)

This classification scheme helps distinguish mildly irritating substances from moderately irritating substances, as well as identifying strongly and severely irritating substances. It is based on the most severe ocular response observed in a group of animals, rather than the average response, and on the persistence of the response.

1. **Nonirritation**

    Exposure of the eye to the material under the specified conditions caused no ocular changes. No tissue staining with fluorescein was observed. Slight conjunctival injection (Grade 1, some vessels definitely injected) that does not clear within 24 hours is not considered a significant change. This level of change is inconsequential as far as representing physical damage to the eye and can be seen to occur naturally for unexplained reasons in otherwise normal rabbits.

2. **Mild Irritation**

    Exposure of the eye to the material under the specified conditions caused minor and/or transient changes as determined by external or slit lamp examination or fluorescein staining. No opacity, ulceration, or fluorescein staining of the cornea (except for staining that is characteristic of normal epithelial desquamation) was observed at any grading interval. The appearance of any of the following changes was sufficient to characterize a response as mild irritation:

    • Grade 1 hyperemia of the iris that is observed at 1 hour, but resolves by 24 hours

    • Grade 2 conjunctival hyperemia that is observed at 1, 24, and/or 48 hours, but resolves by 72 hours

    • Grade 2 conjunctival chemosis that is observed at 1 hour, but diminishes to grade 1 or 0 by 24 hours; or Grade 1 conjunctival chemosis that is observed at 1, and/or 24, and/or 48 hours, but resolves by 72 hours

3. **Moderate Irritation**

    Exposure of the eye to the material under the specified conditions caused major ocular changes as determined by external or slit lamp examination or fluorescein staining. The appearance of any of the following changes was sufficient to characterize a response as moderate irritation:

    • Opacity of the cornea (other than slight dulling of the normal luster) at any observation period, but resolves by day 7

    • Ulceration of the cornea (absence of a confluent patch of corneal epithelium) at any observation period, but resolves by day 7

    • Fluorescein staining of the cornea (greater than that which is characteristic of normal epithelial desquamation) at 1, 2, 3, and/or 4 days, but no staining is found by day 7

    • Grade 1 or 2 hyperemia of the iris (circumcorneal injection) that persists to 24 hours or longer, but resolves by day 7

Table 47   Modified NAS Classification Method Developed by Brendan J. Dunn, Department of Toxicology and Risk Assessment, Honeywell International Inc. (unpublished) (Continued)

- Grade 2 conjunctival hyperemia that persists to at least 72 hours, but resolves by day 7; or Grade 3 conjunctival hyperemia observed at any observation period, but resolves by day 7
- Grade 1 or greater conjunctival chemosis that persists to 72 hours or longer, but resolves by day 7

4.   **Strong Irritation (Clearing within 21 Days)**

Exposure of the eye to the material under the specified conditions resulted in the type of injury described in the former category, but the effects (possibly including pannus or bullae) healed or cleared with 21 days.

5.   **Severe Irritation (Persisting for 21 Days) or Corrosion**

Exposure of the eye to the material under the specified conditions resulted in the type of injury described in the two former categories, but caused significant tissue destruction (necrosis) or injuries that probably adversely affected the visual process. The effects of the injuries persisted for 21 days.

Table 48   Categorization of Substances Using the Slit Lamp Biomicroscope and Fluorescein

Site	"Accept"	"Accept with Caution"	"Probably Injurious to Human Eyes"
Conjunctiva	Hyperemia without chemosis	Chemosis, less than 1 mm at the limbus	Chemosis, greater than 1 mm at the limbus
Cornea	Staining, corneal stippling[a] without confluence at 24 hr	Confluence[b] of staining at 24–48 hr	Staining with infiltration or edema
Anterior chamber	0	0	Flare[c] (visibility of slit beam; rubeosis of iris)

[a]   Corneal stippling: multiple discrete punctate irregularities in the corneal epithelial layer which retain fluorescein.

[b]   Confluence: uniform zones for fluorescein retention larger than 1 mm in diameter.

[c]   Flare: Tyndall effect in a beam traversing the aqueous humor.

Source: From Beckley, J.H., Russell, T.J., and Rubin, L.F. (1969)[5]; U.S. EPA (1988).[6]

Table 49   Categorization and Labeling of Pesticides (Label Statements Regarding Eye Irritation Due to Pesticides)

Toxicity Category	Signal Word	Skull and Crossbones and "Poison" Required	Precautionary Statement	Practical Treatment
I. Corrosive (irreversible destruction of ocular tissue), corneal involvement, or irritation persisting for more than 21 days	Danger	No	Corrosive.[a] Causes irreversible eye damage. Harmful if swallowed. Do not get in eyes or on clothing. Wear (goggles, face shield, or safety glasses).[b] Wash thoroughly with soap and water after handling. Remove contaminated clothing and wash before reuse.	*If in eyes*: flush with plenty of water. Get medical attention. *If swallowed*: promptly drink a large quantity of milk, egg whites, gelatin solution, or, if these are not available, drink large quantities of water. Avoid alcohol. *NOTE TO PHYSICIAN*: Probable mucosal damage may contraindicate the use of gastric lavage.
II. Corneal involvement or irritation clearing in 21 days or less	Warning	No	Causes substantial but temporary eye injury. Do not get into eyes or on clothing. Wear goggles, face shield, or safety glasses.[b] Harmful if swallowed. Wash thoroughly with soap and water after handling. Remove contaminated clothing and wash before reuse.	Same as above; omit *NOTE TO PHYSICIAN* statement.

Table 49   Categorization and Labeling of Pesticides Label Statements Regarding Eye Irritation Due to Pesticides (Continued)

Toxicity Category	Signal Word	Skull and Crossbones and "Poison" Required	Precautionary Statement	Practical Treatment
III. Corneal involvement or irritation clearing in 7 days or less	Caution	No	Causes (moderate) eye injury (irritation). Avoid contact with eyes or clothing. Wash thoroughly with soap and water after handling.	*If in eyes*: Flush with plenty of water. Get medical attention if irritation persists.
IV. Minimal effects clearing in less than 24 hr	Caution	No	None required	None required

a   The term "corrosive" may be omitted if the product is not actually corrosive.

b   Choose appropriate form of eye protection. Recommendation for goggles or face shield is more appropriate for industrial, commercial, or nondomestic uses. Safety glasses may be recommended for domestic or residential use.

Source: From Camp, D.D. (1984).[7]

References

1. Draize, J.H., Woodard, G., and Calvery, H.O., Methods for the study of irritation and toxicity of substances applied topically to the skin and mucous membranes, *J. Pharmacol. Exp. Ter.*, 82, 377, 1944.

2. Kay, J.H. and Calandra, J.C., Interpretation of eye irritation tests, *J. Soc. Cosmet. Chem.*, 13, 281, 1962.

3. Green, W.R. et al., *A Systematic Comparison of Chemically Induced Eye Injury in the Albino Rabbit and Rhesus Monkey*, The Soap and Detergent Association, New York, 1978, 407.

4. Committee for the Revision of NAS Publication 1138, *Principles and Procedures for Evaluating the Toxicity of Household Substances*, National Academy of Sciences, Washington, DC, 1977.

5. Beckley, J.H., Russell, T.J., and Rubin, L.F., Use of the Rhesus monkey for predicting human response to eye irritants, *Toxicol. Appl. Pharmacol.*, 15, 1, 1969.
6. Environmental Protection Agency, Guidance for Evaluation of Eye Irritation Testing, Hazard Evaluation Division Standard Evaluation Procedures, EPA-540/09-88-105, Washington, D.C., 1988.
7. Camp, D.D., *Fed. Reg.*, 49, 188, 1984.

Section 5:
Inhalation Toxicology

Table 50   Body Weight and Lung Volumes in Fischer-344 Rats at Various Ages

Parameter	3 Months	18 Months	27 Months
Body weight (g)	222 ± 61	334 ± 106	332 ± 71
Total lung capacity (TLC) (ml)	11.9 ± 1.7	13.9 ± 2.2	14.4 ± 1.9
TLC/body weight (ml/kg)	56 ± 8	42 ± 7	43 ± 6
Vital capacity (ml)	11.0 ± 1.8	13.4 ± 2.3	13.4 ± 1.7
Functional residual capacity (ml)	2.1 ± 0.3	1.7 ± 0.3	2.7 ± 0.4
Residual volume (RV) (ml)	1.0 ± 0.3	0.6 ± 0.2	1.1 ± 0.5
RV/TLC, (ml/ml)	0.08 ± 0.03	0.04 ± 0.01	0.07 ± 0.03

Note: Values are means ± SD.

Source: Adapted from Mauderly, J.L. (1982).[1] From Sahebjami, H. (1992).[2]

Table 51   Body Weight and Lung Volumes in Adult and Older Hamsters

Parameter	15 Weeks	65 Weeks	*p* Value
Body weight (g)	126 ± 12	125 ± 7	>0.20
Total lung capacity (ml)	9.6 ± 1.3	11.1 ± 1.0	<0.02
Vital capacity (ml)	6.9 ± 1.0	7.8 ± 0.9	<0.10
Functional residual capacity (ml)	3.5 ± 0.5	4.3 ± 0.3	<0.05
Residual volume (RV) (ml)	2.7 ± 0.6	3.3 ± 0.3	<0.05
RV/TLC (%)	28 ± 5	30 ± 5	>0.20

Note: Values are means ± SD.

Source: Adapted from Mauderly, J.L. (1979).[3] From Sahebjami, H. (1992).[2]

Table 52   Ventilatory Parameters in Fischer-344 Rats at Various Ages

Parameter	3 Months	18 Months	27 Months
Respiratory frequency (breath/min)	48 ± 6	54 ± 7	54 ± 6
Tidal volume (ml)	1.1 ± 0.3	1.5 ± 0.3	1.5 ± 0.3
Minute ventilation ($\dot{V}_\varepsilon$) (ml/min)	54 ± 14	82 ± 23	82 ± 18
$\dot{V}_\varepsilon$ body weight (ml/min/kg)	254 ± 48	251 ± 45	252 ± 52

Note: Values are means ± SD.

Source: Adapted from Mauderly, J.L. (1982).[1] From Sahebjami, H. (1992).[2]

Table 53   Ventilatory Parameters in Hamsters at Various Ages

Parameter	15 Weeks	65 Weeks
Respiratory frequency (breath/min)	24 ± 2.7	25 ± 3.9
Tidal volume (ml)	1.2 ± 0.2	1.1 ± 0.2
Minute volume (ml/min)	27.8 ± 3.3	28.1 ± 4.0

Note: Values are means ± SD.

Source: Adapted from Mauderly, J.L. (1979).[3] From Sahebjami, H. (1992).[2]

Table 54   Morphometric Values in Sprague-Dawley Rats at Various Ages

Parameter	4 Months	8 Months	18 Months
V_L body weight (ml/kg)[a]	21.7 ± 1.0	30.9 ± 1.5	38.4 ± 2.8
Lm (μm)[a]	54 ± 2	71 ± 2	87 ± 7
ISA (cm²)	5.571 ± 445[b]	7.979 ± 318	8,733 ± 721

Note: Values are means ± SEM. V_L postfixation lung volume; Lm, mean chord length; ISA, internal surface area.

[a] Significantly different among groups.

[b] Significantly different compared with other groups.

Source: Adapted from Johanson, W.G. Jr. and Pierce, A.K. (1973)[4]; Sahebjami, H. (1992).[2]

Table 55   Normal Cytology of BALF (% of Total Cells)

Animal	Macrophages	Neutro	EOS	Lymph
Rat, mouse, rabbit, Syrian hamster	95	<1	<1	<1
Guinea pig	90	—	10	—
Rabbit	95	<1	<1	4
Dog	85	5	5	5
Sheep	70	5	5	15
Horse	83	5	<1	10
Monkey	89	—	—	10
Human (nonsmoker)	88	<1	<1	10

Note: Abbreviations: BALF = bronchoalveolar lavage fluid; Neutro = neutrophil; EOS = eosinophils; Lymph = lymphocytes.

Source: From Henderson, R.F. (1989).[5] With permission.

Table 56   Normal Biochemical Content of BALF, $\overline{X}$ (SE)

Animal	n	LDH (mlU/ml)	Alkaline Phosphatase (mlU/ml)	Acid Phosphatase (mlU/ml)	β-Glucuronidase (mlU/ml)	Protein (mg/ml)
Rat	240–280	109 (2)	53 (1)	2.4 (0.1)	0.34 (0.02)	0.39 (0.02)
Mouse	45–95	233 (23)	2.5 (0.2)	7.5 (0.8)	0.53 (0.08)	0.82 (0.07)
Guinea pig	6	69 (26)	5.7 (1.6)	2.5 (0.2)	0.65 (0.12)	0.13 (0.03)
Syrian hamster	6	72 (7)	3.6 (1.0)	2.0 (0.1)	0.57 (0.09)	0.37 (0.03)
Rabbit	6	27 (6)	8.5 (4.4)	5.3 (0.5)	0.37 (0.02)	0.44 (0.10)
Dog	4–12	134 (25)	22 (5)	1.4 (0.1)	0.30 (0.04)	0.35 (0.18)
Chimpanzee	5	51 (12)	53 (3)	—	—	0.01 (9.01)

Note: Values are normalized per milliliter of lung volume washed.

Source: From Henderson, R.F. (1989).[5] With permission.

Table 57   Tracheal Mucociliary Clearance

Species	Mucous Velocity[a] (mm/min)
Mouse	+
Rat	1.9 ± 0.7
	5.1 ± 3.0
	5.9 ± 2.5
Ferret	+
	18.2 ± 5.1
	10.7 ± 3.7
Guinea pig	2.7 ± 1.4
Rabbit	3.2 ± 1.1
	+
Chicken	*
Cat	2.5 ± 0.8

Table 57   Tracheal Mucociliary Clearance (Continued)

Species	Mucous Velocity[a] (mm/min)
Dog	21.6 ± 5.0
	9.8 ± 2.1
	19.2 ± 1.6
	7.5 ± 3.7
	14.5 ± 6.3
Baboon	+
Sheep	17.3 ± 6.2
	10.5 ± 2.9
Pig	*
Cow	*
Donkey	14.7 ± 3.8
Horse	16.6 ± 2.4
	17.8 ± 5.1
Human	3.6 ± 1.5
	5.5 ± 0.4
	5.1 ± 2.9
	11.5 ± 4.7
	10.1 ± 3.5
	21.5 ± 5.5
	15.5 ± 1.7

Note: *, transport studied but no velocity given; +, inhalation study, clearance measured but no tracheal velocities given.

[a]   Mean ± SD.

Source: From Wolff, R.K. (1992).[6] With permission.

Table 58   Nasal Mucociliary Clearance

Species	Velocity[a] (mm/min)
Rat	2.3 ± 0.8
Dog	3.7 ± 0.9
Man	5.2 ± 2.3
	5.5 ± 3.2
	5.3 (0.5–23.6)
	8.4 ± 4.8
	6.8 ± 5.1
	7 ± 4

[a] Mean ± SD.

Source: From Wolff, R.K. (1992).[6] With permission.

Table 59   Ammonia Concentrations in an Inhalation Chamber

Animal Loading (%)	Chamber Air Flow (l/min)	No. of Air Changes per Hour	Hour of Sample (ppm NH₃ ± SE)		
			2	4	6
1	13	8	0.38 ± 0.08	0.48 ± 0.07	0.46 ± 0.13
1	26	16	0.20 ± 0.01	0.24 ± 0.02	0.45 ± 0.06
1	40	24	0.19 ± 0.04	0.24 ± 0.05	0.22 ± 0.03
3.1	13	8	0.84 ± 0.14	1.13 ± 0.14	1.11 ± 0.27
3.1	26	16	0.60 ± 0.09	1.04 ± 0.23	1.60 ± 0.22
3.1	40	24	0.19 ± 0.02	0.33 ± 0.05	0.39 ± 0.05
5.1	13	8	1.23 ± 0.18	1.51 ± 0.16	2.42 ± 0.38
5.2	26	16	0.66 ± 0.06	1.23 ± 0.20	2.05 ± 0.41
5.2	40	24	0.46 ± 0.08	1.02 ± 0.11	1.30 ± 0.27

Source: From Phalen, R.F. (1984).[7] With permission.

Table 60 Conversion Table for Gases and Vapors

Molecular Weight	1 mg/l ppm	1 ppm mg/l	Molecular Weight	1 mg/l ppm	1 ppm mg/l	Molecular Weight	1 mg/l ppm	1 ppm mg/l
1	24,450	0.0000409	39	627	0.001595	77	318	0.00315
2	12,230	0.0000818	40	611	0.001636	78	313	0.00319
3	8,150	0.0001227	41	596	0.001677	79	309	0.00323
4	6,113	0.0001636	42	582	0.001718	80	306	0.00327
5	4,890	0.0002045	43	569	0.001759	81	302	0.00331
6	4,075	0.0002454	44	556	0.001800	82	298	0.00335
7	3,493	0.0002863	45	543	0.001840	83	295	0.00339
8	3,056	0.000327	46	532	0.001881	84	291	0.00344
9	2,717	0.000368	47	520	0.001922	85	288	0.00348
10	2,445	0.000409	48	509	0.001963	86	284	0.00352
11	2,223	0.000450	49	499	0.002004	87	281	0.00356
12	2,038	0.000491	50	489	0.002045	88	278	0.00360
13	1,881	0.000532	51	479	0.002086	89	275	0.00364
14	1,746	0.000573	52	470	0.002127	90	272	0.00368
15	1,630	0.000614	53	461	0.002168	91	269	0.00372
16	1,528	0.000654	54	453	0.002209	92	266	0.00376
17	1,438	0.000695	55	445	0.002250	93	263	0.00380
18	1,358	0.000736	56	437	0.002290	94	260	0.00384
19	1,287	0.000777	57	429	0.002331	95	257	0.00389
20	1,223	0.000818	58	422	0.002372	96	255	0.00393
21	1,164	0.000859	59	414	0.002413	97	252	0.00397
22	1,111	0.000900	60	408	0.002554	98	249.5	0.00401
23	1,063	0.000941	61	401	0.002495	99	247.0	0.00405
24	1,019	0.000982	62	394	0.00254	100	244.5	0.00409
25	987	0.001022	63	388	0.00258	101	242.1	0.00413
26	940	0.001063	64	382	0.00262	102	239.7	0.00417
27	906	0.001104	65	376	0.00266	103	237.4	0.00421
28	873	0.001145	66	370	0.00270	104	235.1	0.00425
29	843	0.001186	67	365	0.00274	105	232.9	0.00429
30	815	0.001227	68	360	0.00278	106	230.7	0.00434
31	789	0.001268	69	354	0.00282	107	228.5	0.00438
32	764	0.001309	70	349	0.00286	108	226.4	0.00442
33	741	0.001350	71	344	0.00290	109	224.3	0.00446
34	719	0.001391	72	340	0.00294	110	222.3	0.00450
35	699	0.001432	73	335	0.00299	111	220.3	0.00454
36	679	0.001472	74	330	0.00303	112	218.3	0.00458
37	661	0.001513	75	326	0.00307	113	216.4	0.00462
38	643	0.001554	76	322	0.00311	114	214.5	0.00466

Table 60   Conversion Table for Gases and Vapors (Continued)

Molecular Weight	1 mg/l ppm	1 ppm mg/l	Molecular Weight	1 mg/l ppm	1 ppm mg/l	Molecular Weight	1 mg/l ppm	1 ppm mg/l
115	212.6	0.00470	153	159.8	0.00626	191	128.0	0.00781
116	210.8	0.00474	154	158.8	0.00630	192	127.3	0.00785
117	209.0	0.00479	155	157.7	0.00634	193	126.7	0.00789
118	207.2	0.00483	156	156.7	0.00638	194	126.0	0.00793
119	205.5	0.00487	157	153.7	0.00642	195	125.4	0.00798
120	203.8	0.00491	158	154.7	0.00646	196	124.7	0.00802
121	202.1	0.00495	159	153.7	0.00650	197	124.1	0.00806
122	200.4	0.00499	160	152.8	0.00654	198	123.5	0.00810
123	198.8	0.00503	161	151.9	0.00658	199	122.9	0.00814
124	197.2	0.00507	162	150.9	0.00663	200	122.3	0.00818
125	195.6	0.00511	163	150.0	0.00667	201	121.6	0.00822
126	194.0	0.00515	164	149.1	0.00671	202	121.0	0.00826
127	192.5	0.00519	165	148.2	0.00675	203	120.4	0.00830
128	191.0	0.00524	166	147.3	0.00679	204	119.9	0.00834
129	189.5	0.00528	167	146.4	0.00683	205	119.3	0.00838
130	188.1	0.00532	168	145.5	0.00687	206	118.7	0.00843
131	186.6	0.00536	169	144.7	0.00691	207	118.1	0.00847
132	185.2	0.00540	170	143.8	0.00695	208	117.5	0.00851
133	183.8	0.00544	171	143.0	0.00699	209	117.0	0.00855
134	182.5	0.00548	172	142.2	0.00703	210	116.4	0.00859
135	181.1	0.00552	173	141.3	0.00708	211	115.9	0.00863
136	179.8	0.00556	174	140.5	0.00712	212	115.3	0.00867
137	178.5	0.00560	175	139.7	0.00716	213	114.8	0.00871
138	177.2	0.00564	176	138.9	0.00720	214	114.3	0.00875
139	173.9	0.00569	177	138.1	0.00724	215	113.7	0.00879
140	174.6	0.00573	178	137.4	0.00728	216	113.2	0.00883
141	173.4	0.00577	179	136.6	0.00732	217	112.7	0.00888
142	172.2	0.00581	180	135.8	0.00736	218	112.2	0.00892
143	171.0	0.00585	181	135.1	0.00740	219	111.6	0.00896
144	169.8	0.00589	182	134.3	0.00744	220	111.1	0.00900
145	168.6	0.00593	183	133.6	0.00748	221	110.6	0.00904
146	167.5	0.00597	184	132.9	0.00753	222	110.1	0.00908
147	166.3	0.00601	185	132.2	0.00737	223	109.6	0.00912
148	165.2	0.00605	186	131.5	0.00761	224	109.2	0.00916
149	164.1	0.00609	187	130.7	0.00763	225	108.7	0.00920
150	163.0	0.00613	188	130.1	0.00769	226	108.2	0.00924
151	161.9	0.00618	189	129.4	0.00773	227	107.7	0.00928
152	160.9	0.00622	190	128.7	0.00777	228	107.2	0.00933

Table 60   Conversion Table for Gases and Vapors (Continued)

Molecular Weight	1 mg/l ppm	1 ppm mg/l	Molecular Weight	1 mg/l ppm	1 ppm mg/l	Molecular Weight	1 mg/l ppm	1 ppm mg/l
229	106.8	0.00937	253	96.6	0.01035	277	88.3	0.01133
230	106.3	0.00941	254	96.3	0.01039	278	87.9	0.01137
231	105.8	0.00945	255	95.9	0.01043	279	87.6	0.01141
232	105.4	0.00949	256	95.5	0.01047	280	87.3	0.01145
233	104.9	0.00953	257	95.1	0.01051	281	87.0	0.01149
234	104.3	0.00957	258	94.8	0.01055	282	86.7	0.01153
235	104.0	0.00961	259	94.4	0.01059	283	86.4	0.01157
236	103.6	0.00965	260	94.0	0.01063	284	86.1	0.01162
237	103.2	0.00969	261	93.7	0.01067	285	85.8	0.01166
238	102.7	0.00973	262	93.3	0.01072	286	85.5	0.01170
239	102.3	0.00978	263	93.0	0.01076	287	85.2	0.01174
240	101.9	0.00982	264	92.6	0.01080	288	84.9	0.01178
241	101.5	0.00986	265	92.3	0.01084	289	84.6	0.01182
242	101.0	0.00990	266	91.9	0.01088	290	84.3	0.01186
243	100.6	0.00994	267	91.6	0.01092	291	84.0	0.01190
244	100.2	0.00998	268	91.2	0.01096	292	83.7	0.01194
245	99.8	0.01002	269	90.9	0.01100	293	83.4	0.01198
246	99.4	0.01006	270	90.6	0.01104	294	83.2	0.01202
247	99.0	0.01010	271	90.2	0.01108	295	82.9	0.01207
248	98.6	0.01014	272	89.9	0.01112	296	82.6	0.01211
249	98.2	0.01018	273	89.6	0.01117	297	82.3	0.01215
250	97.8	0.01022	274	89.2	0.01121	298	82.0	0.01219
251	97.4	0.01027	275	88.9	0.01125	299	81.8	0.01223
252	97.0	0.01031	276	88.6	0.01129	300	81.5	0.01227

Source: From Fieldner, A.C., Katz, S.H., and Kinney, S.P. (1921)[8]; Clayton, G.D., and Clayton, F.E., Eds. (1991).[9] With permission.

References

1. Mauderly, J.L., The effect of age on respiratory function of Fischer-344 rats, *Exp. Aging Res.*, 8, 31, 1982.
2. Sahebjami, H., Aging of the normal lung. In *Treatise on Pulmonary Toxicology*, Vol. 1, *Comparative Biology of the Normal Lung*, Parent, R.A., Ed., CRC Press, Boca Raton, FL, 1992, chap. 21.

3. Mauderly, J.L., Ventilation, lung volumes and lung mechanics of young adult and old Syrian hamsters, *Exp. Aging Res.*, 5, 497, 1979.

4. Johanson, W.G., Jr. and Pierce, A.K., Lung structure and function with age in normal rats and rats with papain emphysema, *J. Clin. Invest.*, 52, 2921, 1973.

5. Henderson, R.F., Bronchoalveolar lavage: a tool for assessing the health status of the lung, in *Concepts in Inhalation Toxicology*, McClellan, R.O. and Henderson, R.F., Eds., Hemisphere Publishing, New York, 1989, chap. 15.

6. Wolff, R.K., Mucociliary function, in *Treatise on Pulmonary Toxicology*, Vol. 1, *Comparative Biology of the Normal Lung*, Parent, R.A., Ed., CRC Press, Boca Raton, FL, 1992, chap. 35.

7. Phalen, R.F., *Inhalation Studies: Foundations and Techniques*, CRC Press, Boca Raton, FL, 1984.

8. Fieldner, A.C., Katz, S.H., and Kinney, S.P., Gas Masks for Gasses Met in Fighting Fires, U.S. Bureau of Mines, Tech. Paper No. 248, 1921.

9. Clayton, G.D. and Clayton, F.E., Eds., *Patty's Industrial Hygiene and Toxicology*, 4th ed., John Wiley & Sons, New York, 1991.

Section 6: Neurotoxicology

Table 61   Examples of Potential Endpoints of Neurotoxicity

Behavioral Endpoints
  Absence or altered occurrence, magnitude, or latency of sensorimotor reflex
  Altered magnitude of neurological measurements, such as grip strength or hindlimb splay
  Increases or decreases in motor activity
  Changes in rate or temporal patterning of schedule-controlled behavior
  Changes in motor coordination, weakness, paralysis, abnormal movement or posture, tremor, ongoing performance
  Changes in touch, sight, sound, taste, or smell sensations
  Changes in learning or memory
  Occurrence of seizures
  Altered temporal development of behaviors or reflex responses
  Autonomic signs
Neurophysiological Endpoints
  Change in velocity, amplitude, or refractory period of nerve conduction
  Change in latency or amplitude of sensory-evoked potential
  Change in EEG pattern or power spectrum
Neurochemical Endpoints
  Alteration in synthesis, release, uptake, degradation of neurotransmitters
  Alteration in second messenger-associated signal transduction
  Alteration in membrane-bound enzymes regulating neuronal activity
  Decreases in brain acetylcholinesterase
  Inhibition of neurotoxic esterase
  Altered developmental patterns of neurochemical systems
  Altered proteins (c-fos, substance P)
Structural Endpoints
  Accumulation, proliferation, or rearrangement of structural elements
  Breakdown of cells
  GFAP increases (adults)
  Gross changes in morphology, including brain weight
  Discoloration of nerve tissue
  Hemorrhage in nerve tissue

Source: From U.S. EPA (1993).[1]

Table 62 Examples of Parameters Recorded in Neurotoxicity Safety Studies

Clinical signs of neurotoxicity (onset and duration)
Body weight changes
Changes in behavior
Observations of skin, eyes, mucous membranes, etc.
Signs of autonomic nervous system effect (e.g., tearing, salivation, diarrhea)
Changes in respiratory rate and depth
Cardiovascular changes such as flushing
Central nervous system changes such as tremors, convulsion, or coma
Time of death
Necropsy results
Histopathological findings of the brain, spinal cord, and peripheral nerves

Source: From Abou-Donia, M.B. (1992).[2]

Table 63 Summary of Measures in the Functional Observational Battery and the Type of Data Produced by Each

Home Cage and Open Field	Manipulative	Physiological
Posture (D)	Ease of removal (R)	Body temperature (I)
Convulsions, tremors (D)	Handling reactivity (R)	Body weight (I)
Palpebral closure (R)	Palpebral closure (R)	
Lacrimation (R)	Approach response (R)	
Piloerection (Q)	Click response (R)	
Salivation (R)	Touch response (R)	
Vocalizations (Q)	Tail pinch response (R)	
Rearing (C)	Righting reflex (R)	
Urination (C)	Landing foot play (I)	
Defecation (C)	Forelimb grip-strength (I)	
Gait (D,R)	Hindlimb grip-strength (I)	
Arousal (R)	Pupil response (Q)	
Mobility (R)		
Stereotype (D)		
Bizarre behavior (D)		

Note: D, descriptive data; R, rank order data; Q, quantal data; I, interval data; C, count data.

Source: From U.S. EPA (1993).[1]

Table 64   Examples of Organophosphorus Pesticides Producing Delayed Neuropathy

Compound	Hen (mg/kg)	Human Cases
Mipafox	25 IM	2
Haloxon	1000 PO	—
EPN	40–80 SC	3
Trichlornat	310 PO	2
Leptophos	400–500 PO	8
Desbromoleptophos	60 PO	—
DEF	1110 SC	—
Cyanofenphos	>100 PO	—
Isofenphos	100 PO	—
Dichlorvos	100 SC	—
Amiprophos	600 PO	—
Coumaphos	50 PO	—
Chlorpyrifos	150 PO	1
Salithion	120 PO	—
Methaminophos	—	9
Trichlorphon	—	Many

Source: Adapted from Environmental Health Criteria, World Health Organization (1986).[3]

References

1. U.S. Environmental Protection Agency, Draft Report: Principles of Neurotoxicity Risk Assessment, *Chemical Regulation Reporter*, Bureau of National Affairs, Inc., Washington D.C., 1993, 900–943.
2. Abou-Donia, M.B., Principles and methods of evaluating neurotoxicity, in *Neurotoxicology*, Abou-Donia, M.B., Ed., CRC Press, Boca Raton, FL, 1992, 515.
3. Environmental Health Criteria, *Organophosphorus Insecticides: A General Introduction*, World Health Organization, Geneva, 1986, 6.

Section 7: Immunotoxicology

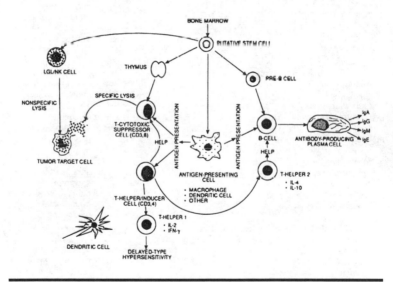

Figure 1   Cellular elements of the immune system.

Table 65   Examples of the Four Types of Hypersensitivity Responses

Agents: Clinical Manifestations	Hypersensitive Reaction	Cells Involved	Antibody	Mechanism of Cell Injury
Food additives: GI allergy Penicillin: urticaria and dermatitis	Type I (anaphylactic)	Mast cell	IgE (and others)	Degranulation and release of inflammatory mediators such as histamine, proteolytic enzymes, chemotactic factors, prostaglandins, and leukotrienes
Cephalosporins: hemolytic anemia Aminopyrine: leukopenia Quinidine, gold: thrombocytopenia	Type II (cytotoxic)	Null (K) cells[a]	IgG, IgM	Antibody-dependent cellular cytotoxicity, or complement-mediated lysis
Hydralazine: systemic lupus erythomatosis Methicillin: chronic glomerulonephritis	Type III (immune complex)	PMNs[b]	IgG, IgM	Immune complex deposition in various tissues activates complement, which attracts PMNs causing local damage by release of inflammatory mediators
Nickel, penicillin, dinitrochloro-benzene, phenothiasines: contact dermatitis	Type IV (delayed hypersensitivity)	T cells (sensitized); macrophages	None	Release of lymphokines activates and attracts macrophages, which release mediators that induce inflammatory reactions

Note: Defined by Coombs and Gell (1968).[1]

[a]   Also T cells, monocyte/macrophages, platelets, neutrophils, and eosinophils.

[b]   Polymorphonuclear leukocytes.

Source: From Norbury, K. and Thomas P. (1990).[2] With permission.

Table 66   Examples of Antemortem and Postmortem Findings that May Include Potential Immunotoxicity if Treatment Related

Parameter	Possible Observation (Cause)	Possible State of Immune Competence
Antemortem		
Mortality	Increased (infection)	Depressed
Body weight	Decreased (infection)	Depressed
Clinical signs	Rales, nasal discharge (respiratory infection)	Depressed
	Swollen cervical area (sislodacryoadenitis virus)	Depressed
Physical examinations	Enlarged tonsils (infection)	Depressed
Hematology	Leukopenia/lymphopenia	Depressed
	Leukocytosis (infection/cancer)	Enhanced/depressed
	Thrombocytopenia	Hypersensitivity
	Neutropenia	Hypersensitivity
Protein electrophoresis	Hypogammaglobulinemia	Depressed
	Hypergammaglobulinemia (ongoing immune response or infection)	Enhanced/activated
Postmortem		
Organ weights		
Thymus	Decreased	Depressed
Histopathology		
Adrenal glands	Cortical hypertrophy (stress)	Depressed (secondary)
Bone marrow	Hypoplasia	Depressed
Kidney	Amyloidosis	Autoimmunity
	Glomerulonephritis (immune complex)	Hypersensitivity
Lung	Pneumonitis (infection)	Depressed
Lymph node (see also spleen)	Atrophy	Depressed
Spleen	Hypertrophy/hyperplasia	Enhanced/activated
	Depletion of follicles	Depressed B cells
	Hypocellularity of periarteriolar sheath	Depressed T cells
	Active germinal centers	Enhanced/activated
Thymus	Atrophy	Depressed
Thyroid	Inflammation	Autoimmunity

Source: From Norbury, K. and Thomas, P. (1990).[2] With permission.

Table 67   U.S. EPA Subdivision M Guidelines for Immunotoxicity Testing of Biochemical Pest Control Agents (BPCA)

I. Tier I

A.   Spleen, thymus, and bone marrow cellularity.

B.   Humoral Immunity — do one of the following:
1.   Primary and secondary immunoglobulin (IgG and IgM) responses to antigen; or,
2.   Antibody plaque-forming cell assay.

C.   Specific cell-mediated immunity — do one of the following:
1.   One-way mixed lymphocyte reaction (MLR) assay; or,
2.   Delayed-type hypersensitivity (DTH) assay; or,
3.   Cytotoxic T-lymphocyte (CTL) assay.

D.   Nonspecific cell-mediated immunity:
1.   Natural killer cell activity; and,
2.   Macrophage function.

II. Tier II

A.   Tier II studies required if:
1.   Dysfunction is observed in Tier I tests.
2.   Tier I test results cannot be definitively interpreted.
3.   Data from other sources indicate immunotoxicity.

B.   General testing features:
1.   Evaluate time course for recovery from immunotoxic effects.
2.   Determine whether observed effects may impair host resistance to infectious agents or to tumor cell challenge.
3.   Perform additional specific, but appropriate, testing essential for evaluation of potential risks.

Source: Adapted from Sjoblad, R. (1988).[3]

Table 68   National Toxicology Program Panel for Detecting Immune Alterations in Rodents

Parameter	Procedures
	Screen (Tier I)
Immunopathology	• Hematology: Complete blood count and differential
	• Weights: Body, spleen, thymus, kidney, liver
	• Cellularity: Spleen
	• Histology: Spleen, thymus, lymph node
Humoral immunity	• Enumerate IgM antibody plaque-forming cells to T-dependent antigen (sRBC)
	• LPS mitogen response
Cell-mediated immunity	• Lymphocyte blastogenesis to mitogens (Con A)
	• Mixed leukocyte response against allogeneic leukocytes (MLR)
Nonspecific immunity	• Natural killer (NK) cell activity
	Comprehensive (Tier II)
Immunopathology	• Quantitation of splenic B and T cell numbers
Humoral-mediated immunity	• Enumeration of IgG antibody response to sRBCs
Cell-mediated immunity	• Cytotoxic T lymphocyte (CTL) cytolysis
	• Delayed hypersensitivity response (DHR)
Nonspecific immunity	• Macrophage function-quantitation of resident peritoneal cells, and phagocytic ability (basal and activated by MAF)
Host resistance challenge models (endpoints)[a]	• Syngeneic tumor cells
	• PYB6 sarcoma (tumor incidence)
	• B16F10 melanoma (lung burden)
	• Bacterial models: *Listeria monocytogenes; Streptococcus species*
	• Viral models: Influenza
	• Parasite models: *Plasmodium yoelii* (Parasitaemia)

Note: The testing panel was developed using B6C3F1 female mice.

[a]   For any particular chemical tested, only two or three host resistance models are selected for examination.

Source: Adapted from Luster, M.I., Portier, C., Pait, D., Whilte, K., Genning, C., Munson, A., and Rosenthal, G. (1992).[4]

References

1. Coombs, R.R.A. and Gell, P.G.H., Classification of allergic reactions responsible for clinical hypersensitivity and disease, in *Clinical Aspects of Immunology*, Gell, P. and Coombs, R., Eds., Blackwell Scientific, Oxford, 1968, 121–137.
2. Norbury, K. and Thomas, P., Assessment of immunotoxicity, in *In vivo Toxicity Testing: Principles, Procedures and Practices*, Arnold, D.L., Grice, H., and Krewski, D., Eds., Academic Press, New York, 1990, 410–448.
3. Sjoblad, R., Potential future requirements for immunotoxicology testing of pesticides, *Toxicol. Indust. Health*, 4, 391–395, 1988.
4. Luster, M.I., Portier, C., Pait, D., Whilte, K., Genning, C., Munson, A., and Rosenthal, G., Risk assessment in immunotoxicology I. Sensitivity and predictability of immune tests, *Fundam. Appl. Toxicol.*, 18, 200–210, 1992.

Section 8: Carcinogenesis

Table 69   Characteristics of Initiation, Promotion, and Progression

Initiation	Promotion	Progression
• Irreversible	• Reversible	• Irreversible
• Additive	• Nonadditive	• Karyotypic abnormalities appear accompanied by increased growth rate and invasiveness
• Dose response can be demonstrated; does not exhibit a readily measurable threshold	• Dose response having a measurable threshold can be demonstrated	• Benign and/or malignant tumor observed
• No measurable maximum response	• Measurable maximum effect	• Environmental factors influence early stage of progression
• Initiators are usually genotoxic	• Promoters are usually not mutagenic	• Progressors may not be initiators
• One exposure may be sufficient	• Prolonged and repeated exposure to promoters required	• Progressors act to advance promoted cells to a potentially malignant stage
• Must occur prior to promotion	• Promoter effective only after initiation has occurred	• Spontaneous progression can occur
• Requires fixation through cell division	• Promoted cell population dependent on continued presence of promoter	
• Initiated cells are not identifiable except as foci lesions following a period of promotion	• Causes expansion of the progeny of initiated cells producing foci lesions	
• "Pure" initiation does not result in neoplasia without promotion	• "Pure" promoters not capable of initiation	
• Spontaneous (fortuitous) initiation can occur	• Sensitive to hormonal and dietary factors	

Source: Adapted from Pitot, H.C. (1991)[1] and Maronpot, R.R. (1991).[2]

Table 70   Classification of Carcinogenic Chemicals Based on Mode of Action

	Classification[a]	Mode of Action	Examples
I.	Genotoxic	Agents which interact with DNA.	
	1. Direct acting (primary carcinogen; activation-independent)	Organic chemicals; direct alteration of DNA, chromosome structure or number, metabolic conversion not required; generation of reactive electrophiles and covalent binding to DNA.	Bischloromethylether, β-propiolactone, ethylene imine
	2. Procarcinogen (secondary carcinogen; activation-dependent)	Organic chemicals; requires biotransformation to a direct-acting carcinogen (proximate carcinogen).	Nitrosamines, ethylene dibromide, vinyl chloride
	3. Inorganic carcinogen	Direct effects on DNA may occur through interference with DNA replication.	Nickel, cadmium
II.	Epigenetic	Agents for which there is no direct evidence of interaction with DNA.	
	4. Cytotoxin	Cytolethal; induction of regenerative cell proliferation; mutations may occur secondarily through several mechanisms, including: release of nucleases, generation of reactive oxygen radicals, DNA replication before adduct repair; preferential growth of preneoplastic cells may be caused by selective killing of normal cells or expression of growth control genes (oncogenes).	Nitrilo triacetic acid, chloroform
	5. Mitogen	Stimulation of mitogeneic cell proliferation directly or via a cellular receptor; mutations may occur secondarily as a result of increased cell proliferation; preferential growth of preneoplastic cells may be caused through alteration of rates of cell birth or death.	Phenobarbital, α-hexachloro-cyclohexane

Table 70   Classification of Carcinogenic Chemicals Based on Mode of Action (Continued)

	Classification[a]	Mode of Action	Examples
6.	Peroxisome proliferator	Generation of reactive oxygen radicals through pertubation of lipid metabolism; growth control genes may be activated directly or via a cellular receptor.	Fenofibrate, diethylhexyl phthalate, clofibrate
7.	Immunosuppressor	Enhancement of the development of virally induced, transplanted and metastatic neoplasms, possibly through impairment or loss of natural and acquired tumor resistance.	Azathioprine, cyclosporin A, 6-mercaptopurine
8.	Hormones and hormonal-altering agents	Chronic stimulation of cell growth through activation of regulatory genes; other potential modes of action include: promotional effects resulting from alteration of hormonal homeostasis, inhibition of cell death (apoptosis), generation of reactive radicals.	Estrogens, diethylstilbestrol, synthetic androgens
9.	Solid-state carcinogen	Generally only mesenchymal cells/tissues affected; physical size and shape of agent is critical; mechanism of action uncertain.	Polymers (plastic), metal foils (gold), asbestos
10.	Cocarcinogen	*Simultaneous* administration enhances the carcinogenic process caused by a genotoxic carcinogen; possible mechanisms include: enhanced biotransformation of a procarcinogen, inhibition of detoxification of a primary carcinogen, enhanced absorption or decreased elimination of a genotoxic carcinogen.	Phorbol esters, catechol, ethanol

Table 70   Classification of Carcinogenic Chemicals Based on Mode of Action (Continued)

	Classification[a]	Mode of Action	Examples
11.	Promoter	Administration *subsequent* to a genotoxic agent promotes tumor formation through enhancement of the clonal expansion of preneoplastic cells; multiple and diverse mechanisms proposed.	Phorbol esters, saccharin, croton oil
12.	Progressor	Development of initiated/promoted cells influenced; associated with alterations in biochemical and morphological characteristics, increased growth rate, invasiveness, and metastases; direct or indirect induction of structural (karyotypic) changes to chromosomes.	Arsenic salts, benzene, hydoxyurea

[a] Classifications shown are not rigid. For example, a chemical may be both genotoxic and mitogenic or cytotoxic; phorbol ester can be both a promoter and a cocarcinogen.

Source: Adapted from Weisburger, J.H. and Williams, G.M. (1980).[3] *Additional sources*: Pitot, H.C. and Dragon, Y.P. (1993)[4]; Pitot, H.C. (1993)[5]; Maronpot, R.R. (1991)[2]; and Butterworth, B.E. and Goldsworthy, T.L. (1991).[6]

Table 71   Reported Percent Incidence (Range) of Spontaneous Tumor Formation in Various Mouse Strains

Organ/Tissue	CD-1		B6C3F1	
	Male	Female	Male	Female
Adrenal	0–27.9(%)	0–38	<1.0–1.4	<1.0
Body cavities	—	—	<1.0	<1.0
Brain	—	0–2.0	<0.1–0.1	0–0.1
Circulatory system	—	—	<1.0–2.9	<1.0–2.4
Heart	—	—	0.1–<1.0	0–0.1
Intestines	—	—	<1.0	<1.0
Kidney	0–2.8	0–1.4	<1.0	<0.1–<1.0
Leukemia/ lymphoma	0–8.6	1.4–25.0	1.6–19.0	1.7–33.2
Liver	0–17.3	0–7.1	15.6–40.1	2.5–10.5
Lung/trachea	0–26.0	0–38.6	9.2–22.5	3.5–7.1
Mammary gland	—	0–7.3	—	<1.0–1.3
Ovary	NA	0–4.8	NA	<1.0
Pancreas	—	—	0.1–2.1	<0.1–<1.0
Pancreatic islets	0–2.1	0–1.4	<1.0	<1.0
Pituitary	0–0.8	0–10.0	<1.0	3.2–13.1
Skin/subcutaneous	0–2.8	0–2.0	<0.1–1.9	0.1–1.6
Stomach	0–4.9	0–3.8	0.3–1.1	<1.0
Testes[a]	0–2.0	NA	<1.0	NA
Thyroid	0–2.0	—	1.0–1.1	<1.0–1.7
Urinary bladder	0–2.0	0–1.4	0–0.1	<0.1–1.0
Uterus/vagina	NA	0–13.3	NA	1.2–1.9

[a]   Includes prostate and seminal vesicles.

Source: Adapted from Gad, S.C. and Weil, C.S. (1986).[7] *Additional sources*: Chu, K. (1977)[8]; Fears, T.R., Tarone, R.E., and Chu, K.C. (1977)[9]; Page, N.P. (1977)[10]; Gart, J.J., Chu, K.C., and Tarone, R.E. (1979)[11]; Tarone, R.E., Chu, K.C., and Ward, J.M. (1981)[12]; Rao, G.N., Haseman, J.K., Grumbein, S., Crawford, D.D., and Eustis, S.L. (1990)[13]; and Lang, P.L. (1987).[14]

Table 72   Reported Percent Incidence (Range) of Spontaneous Tumor Formation in Various Rat Strains

Organ/Tissue	F-344 Male	F-344 Female	Sprague-Dawley Male	Sprague-Dawley Female	Wistar Male	Wistar Female
Adrenal	2.4–38.1(%)	4.0–12.0	1.4–7.6	2.7–4.3	0–48.6	0–57.1
Body cavities	<1.0–9.0	0.3–1.9	1.1–1.4	1.8	—	—
Brain	0.8–8.1	<1.0	1.4–2.7	0.9–1.6	0–8.0	0–6.0
Circulatory system	0.4–3.8	<1.0	0.5	—	—	—
Heart	<1.0	<1.0	—	—	0	0
Intestines	<1.0	<1.0	—	0.5	0–2.0	0–2.1
Kidney	<1.0	<1.0	1.6	0.9	0–2.0	0–2.0
Leukemia/ lymphoma	6.5–48.0	2.1–24.6	1.9–2.2	1.4–1.6	0–12.0	0–16.0
Liver	0.5–3.4	0.5–3.9	1.1	0.5–2.2	0–2.5	0–12.0
Lung/trachea	<1.0–3.0	<1.0–2.0	1.6	2.2	0–5.7	0–2.1
Mammary gland	0–1.5	8.5–41.0	0.5–2.3	36.4–45.1	0–4.0	1.3–24.0
Ovary	NA	<1.0	NA	1.1	NA	0–4.3
Pancreas	0.2–6.0	0	—	—	—	—
Pancreatic islets	0.8–4.9	0.8–1.3	0.9–2.7	0.5	0–5.9	0–4.0
Pituitary	4.7–34.7	0.3–58.6	11.2–33.2	37.3–57.6	2.3–58.3	6.7–68.0
Preputial gland	1.4–2.4	1.2–1.8	—	—	—	—
Skin/ subcutaneous	5.7–7.8	2.5–3.2	2.8–6.5	3.2–3.8	0–12.0	0–4.0
Stomach	<1.0	<1.0	—	—	0	0–2.2
Testes[a]	2.3–90.0	NA	4.2–4.3	NA	0–22.0	NA
Thyroid	3.6–12.0	4.7–10.0	1.9–3.8	1.8	0–19.3	2.5–22.4
Urinary bladder	<1.0	<1.0	0.5	—	0–2.0	0–2.0
Uterus/vagina	NA	5.5–24.6	NA	3.3–4.5	NA	1.1–25.3

[a]   Includes prostate and seminal vesicles.

Source: Adapted from Gad, S.C. and Weil, C.S. (1986).[7] *Additional sources*: Chu, K. (1977)[8]; Fears, T.R., Tarone, R.E., and Chu, K.C. (1977)[9]; Page, N.P. (1977)[10]; Gart, J.J., Chu, K.C., and Tarone, R.E. (1979)[11]; Tarone, R.E., Chu, K.C., and Ward, J.M. (1981)[12]; Goodman, D.G., Ward, J.M., Squire, R.A., Chu, K.C., and Linhart, M.S. (1979)[15]; Bombard, E., Karbe, E., and Loeser, E. (1986)[16]; Walsh, K.M. and Poteracki, J., (1994)[17]; Haseman, J.K. (1983)[18]; and Rao, G.N., Haseman, J.K., Brumbein, S., Crawford, D.D., and Eustis, S.L. (1990).[19]

Table 73 Frequency of Carcinogenic Response to Chemicals by Organ/System — Rats and Mice

	Number Positive at Site (%)[a]	
	Chemicals Evaluated as Carcinogenic in Rats ($n = 354$)[b]	Chemicals Evaluated as Carcinogenic in Mice ($n = 299$)[b]
Liver	143 (40%)	171 (57%)
Lung	31 (9%)	83 (28%)
Mammary gland	73 (21%)	14 (5%)
Stomach	60 (17%)	42 (14%)
Vascular system	26 (7%)	47 (16%)
Kidney/ureter	45 (13%)	12 (4%)
Hematopoietic system	35 (10%)	39 (13%)
Urinary bladder/urethra	37 (10%)	12 (4%)
Nasal cavity/turbinates	33 (9%)	4 (1%)
Ear/Zymbal's gland	30 (9%)	2
Esophagus	29 (8%)	7 (2%)
Small intestine	21 (6%)	3 (1%)
Thyroid gland	20 (6%)	10 (3%)
Skin	20 (6%)	1
Peritoneal cavity	17 (5%)	7 (2%)
Oral cavity	16 (5%)	1
Large intestine	15 (4%)	
Central nervous system	15 (4%)	2
Uterus	11 (3%)	5 (2%)
Subcutaneous tissue	10 (3%)	1
Pancreas	9 (3%)	
Adrenal gland	7 (2%)	4 (1%)
Pituitary gland	7 (2%)	4 (1%)
Clitoral gland	7 (2%)	2
Preputial gland	2	7 (2%)
Testes	6 (2%)	1
Harderian gland		6 (2%)
Spleen	6 (2%)	
Ovary		4 (1%)
Gall bladder		3 (1%)
Bone	3	

Table 73　Frequency of Carcinogenic Response to Chemicals by Organ/System — Rats and Mice (Continued)

	Number Positive at Site (%)[a]	
	Chemicals Evaluated as Carcinogenic in Rats ($n = 354$)[b]	Chemicals Evaluated as Carcinogenic in Mice ($n = 299$)[b]
Mesovarium	2	
Myocardium		2
Prostrate	2	
Vagina	1	

Note: Based on 354 and 299 chemicals considered carcinogenic to rats and mice, respectively, in long-term chemical carcinogenesis studies from the carcinogenic potency database (CPDB).

[a]　Percentages not given when fewer than 1% of the carcinogens were active at a given site.

[b]　Chemicals have been excluded for which the only positive results in the CPDB are for "all tumor-bearing animals," i.e., there is no reported target site.

Source: From Gold, L.S., Slone, T.H., Manley, N.B., and Bernstein, L. (1991).[20]

Table 74   Capacity of Tissues to Undergo Hyperplasia

High capacity
  Surface epithelium
  Hepatocytes
  Renal tubules
  Fibroblasts
  Endothelium
  Mesothelium
  Hematopoietic stem cells
  Lymphoid cells

Moderate capacity
  Glandular epithelium
  Bone
  Cartilage
  Smooth muscle of vessels
  Smooth muscle of uterus

Low capacity
  Neurons
  Skeletal muscle
  Smooth muscle of GI tract

Source: From Maronpot, R.R. (1991).[2]
With permission.

Table 75 Selected Examples of Presumptive Preneoplastic Lesions

Tissue	Presumptive Preneoplastic Lesion[a]
Mammary gland	Hyperplastic alveolar nodules (HANs)
	Atypical epithelial proliferation
	Lobular hyperplasia
	Intraductal hyperplasia
	Hyperplastic terminal duct
Liver	Foci of cellular alteration
	Hepatocellular hyperplasia
	Oval cell proliferation
	Cholangiofibrosis
Kidney	Karyocytomegaly
	Atypical tubular dilation
	Atypical tubular hyperplasia
Skin	Increase in dark basal keratinocytes
	Focal hyperplasia/hyperkeratosis
Pancreas (exocrine)	Foci of acinar cell alteration
	Hyperplastic nodules
	Atypical acinar cell nodules

[a] Many of these presumptive preneoplastic lesions are seen in carcinogenicity studies utilizing specific animal model systems. Generalizations about these presumptive preneoplastic lesions are inappropriate outside the context of the specific animal model system being used.

Source: From Maronpot, R.R. (1991).[2] With permission.

Table 76   Comparative Features of Benign and Malignant Neoplasms

	Benign	Malignant
General effect on the host	Little; usually do not cause death	Will almost always kill the host if untreated.
Rate of growth	Slow; may stop or regress	More rapid (but slower than "repair" tissue); autonomous; never stop or regress
Histologic features	Encapsulated; remain localized at primary site	Infiltrate or invade; metastasize
Mode of growth	Usually grow by expansion, displacing surrounding normal tissue	Invade, destroy, and replace surrounding normal tissue
Metastasis	Do not metastasize	Most can metastasize
Architecture	Encapsulated; have complex stroma and adequate blood supply	Not encapsulated; usually have poorly developed stroma; may become necrotic at center
Danger to host	Most without lethal significance	Always ultimately lethal unless removed or destroyed *in situ*
Injury to host	Usually negligible but may become very large and compress or obstruct vital tissue	Can kill host directly by destruction of vital tissue
Radiation sensitivity	Radiation sensitivity near that of normal parent cell; rarely treated with radiation	Radiation sensitivity increased in rough proportion to malignancy; often treated with radiation.
Behavior in tissue	Cells cohesive and inhibited by mutual contact	Cells do not cohere, frequently not inhibited by mutual contact
Resemblance to tissue origin	Cells and architecture resemble tissue of origin	Cells atypical and pleomorphic; disorganized bizarre architecture
Mitotic figures	Mitotic figures rare and normal	Mitotic figures may be numerous and abnormal in polarity and configuration
Shape of nucleus	Normal and regular, show usual stain affinity	Irregular; nucleus frequently hyperchromatic
Size of nucleus	Normal; ratio of nucleus to cytoplasm near normal	Frequently large; nucleus to cytoplasm ratio increased
Nucleolus	Not conspicuous	Hyperchromatic and larger than normal

Source: From Maronpot, R.R. (1991).[2] With permission.

Table 77   Selected Taxonomy of Neoplasia

Tissue	Benign Neoplasia[a]	Malignant Neoplasia[b]
Epithelium		
Squamous	Squamous cell papilloma	Squamous cell carcinoma
Transitional	Transitional cell papilloma	Transitional cell carcinoma
Glandular		
Liver cell	Hepatocellular adenoma	Hepatocellular carcinoma
Islet cell	Islet cell adenoma	Islet cell adenocarcinoma
Connective tissue		
Adult fibrous	Fibroma	Fibrosarcoma
Embryonic fibrous	Myxoma	Myxosarcoma
Cartilage	Chondroma	Chondrosarcoma
Bone	Osteoma	Osteosarcoma
Fat	Lipoma	Liposarcoma
Muscle		
Smooth muscle	Leiomyoma	Leiomyosarcoma
Skeletal muscle	Rhabdomyoma	Rhabdomyosarcoma
Cardiac muscle	Rhabdomyoma	Rhabdomyosarcoma
Endothelium		
Lymph vessels	Lymphangioma	Lymphangiosarcoma
Blood vessels	Hemangioma	Hemangiosarcoma
Lymphoreticular		
Thymus	(not recognized)	Thymoma
Lymph nodes	(not recognized)	Lymphosarcoma (malignant lymphoma)
Hematopoietic		

Bone marrow	(not recognized)	Leukemia
		    Granulocytic
		    Monocytic
		    Erythroleukemia

Neural tissue		
Nerve sheath	Neurilemmona	Neurogenic sarcoma
Glioma	Glioma	Malignant glioma
Astrocytes	Astrocytoma	Malignant astrocytoma
Embryonic cells	(not recognized)	Neuroblastoma

[a] "-oma," benign neoplasm.

[b] "Sarcoma," malignant neoplasm of mesenchymal origin, "carcinoma," malignant neoplasm of epithelial origin.

Source: From Maronpot, R.R. (1991).[2] With permission.

References

1. Pitot, H.C., Endogenous carcinogenesis: the role of tumor promotion, *Proc. Soc. Exp. Biol. Med.*, 198, 661, 1991.

2. Maronpot, R.R., Chemical carcinogenesis, in *Handbook of Toxicologic Pathology*, Haschek, W.M. and Rousseaux, G.G., Eds., Academic Press, San Diego, 1991, chap. 7.

3. Weisburger, J.H. and Williams, G.M., Chemical carcinogens, in *Cassarett and Doull's Toxicology: The Basic Science of Poisons*, 2nd ed., Doull, J., Klaassen, C.D., and Amdur, M.O., Eds., Macmillan, New York, 1980, chap. 6.

4. Pitot, H.C. and Dragon, Y.P., Stage of tumor progression, progressor agents, and human risk, *Proc. Soc. Exp. Biol. Med.*, 202, 37, 1993.

5. Pitot, H.C., The dynamics of carcinogenesis: implications for human risk, *C.I.I.T. Activities*, Chemical Industry Institute of Toxicology, Vol. 13, No. 6, 1993.

6. Butterworth, B.E. and Goldsworthy, T.L., The role of cell proliferation in multistage carcinogenesis, *Proc. Soc. Exp. Biol. Med.*, 198, 683, 1991.

7. Gad, S.C. and Weil, C.S., *Statistics and Experimental Design for Toxicologists*, Telford Press, New Jersey, 1986.

8. Chu, K., *Percent Spontaneous Primary Tumors in Untreated Species Used at NCI for Carcinogen Bioassays*, NCI Clearing House, 1977; as cited in Gad and Weil.[7]

9. Fears, T.R., Tarone, R.E., and Chu, K.C., False-positive and false-negative rates for carcinogenicity screens, *Cancer Res.*, 27, 1941, 1977; as cited in Gad and Weil.[7]

10. Page, N.P., Concepts of a bioassay program in environmental carcinogenesis, in *Environmental Cancer*, Kraybill, H.F. and Mehlman, M.A., Eds., Hemisphere Publishing, New York, 1977, 87-171; as cited in Gad and Weil.[7]

11. Gart, J.J., Chu, K.C., and Tarone, R.E., Statistical issues in interpretation of chronic bioassay tests for carcinogenicity, *J. Natl. Cancer Inst.*, 62, 957, 1979; as cited in Gad and Weil.[7]

12. Tarone, R.E., Chu, K.C., and Ward, J.M., Variability in the rates of some common naturally occurring tumors in Fischer 344 rats and (C57BL/6NXC3H/HEN) F' (B6C3F₁) mice, *J. Natl. Cancer Inst.*, 66, 1175, 1981; as cited in Gad and Weil.[7]

13. Rao, G.N., Haseman, J.K., Grumbein, S., Crawford, D.D., and Eustis, S.L., Growth, body weight, survival and tumor trends in (C57BL/6 X C3H/HeN)F₁ (B6C3F1) mice during a nine-year period, *Toxicol. Pathol.*, 18, 71, 1990.

14. Lang, P.L., Spontaneous Neoplastic Lesions in the Crl:CD-1®(ICR)BR Mouse, Charles River Laboratories, Wilmington, MA, 1987.

15. Goodman, D.G., Ward, J.M., Squire, R.A., Chu, K.C., and Linhart, M.S., Neoplastic and nonneoplastic lesions in aging F344 rats, *Toxicol. Appl. Pharmacol.*, 48, 237, 1979; as cited in Gad and Weil.[7]

16. Bombard, E., Karbe, E., and Loeser, E., Spontaneous tumors of 2000 Wistar TNO/W.70 rats in two-year carcinogenicity studies, *J. Environ. Pathol. Toxicol. Oncol.*, 7, 35, 1986.

17. Walsh, K.M. and Poteracki, J., Spontaneous neoplasms in control Wistar rats, *Fundam. Appl. Toxicol.*, 22, 65, 1994.

18. Haseman, J.K., Patterns of tumor incidence in two-year cancer bioassay feeding studies in Fischer 344 rats, *Fundam. Appl. Toxicol.*, 3, 1, 1983.

19. Rao, G.N., Haseman, J.K., Grumbein, S., Crawford, D.D., and Eustis, S.L., Growth, body weight, survival and tumor trends in F344/N rats during an eleven-year period, *Toxicol. Pathol.*, 18, 61, 1990.

20. Gold, L.S., Slone, T.H., Manley, N.B., and Bernstein, L., Target organs in chronic bioassays of 533 chemical carcinogens, *Environ. Health Perspect.*, 93, 233, 1991.

Section 9:
Reproductive/
Developmental Toxicology

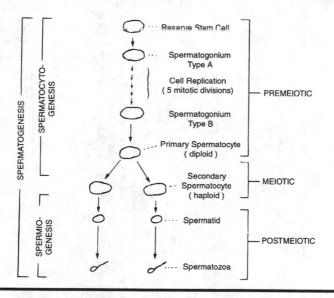

Figure 2   A general scheme of mammalian spermatogenesis, showing the premeiotic and meiotic stages of spermatocytogenesis (from reserve stem cells through the primary diploid spermatocyte to the haploid secondary spermatocyte) and the postmeiotic spermiogenesis with the development and maturation of the spermatozoa. Each cycle is completed in 35 to 64 days, depending on the species, with a new cycle being initiated at the Type A spermatogonium level every 12 to 13 days. (From Ecobichon, D.J., *The Basis of Toxicity Testing,* **CRC Press, Boca Raton, FL, 1992, chap. 5, Fig. 2.)[1]**

Table 78   Breeding Characteristics of Female Laboratory Mammals Compared with the Human

Parameters	Monkey[b]	Dog	Cat	Rabbit	Mouse	Guinea Pig	Hamster	Rat	Human
Age at puberty (days)	36 mo	6–8 mo	6–15 mo	5.5–8.5 mo	35 d	55–70 d	35–56 d	37–67 d	12–15 yr
Breeding season	Oct.–Jan.	Spring–Fall	Feb.–July	All year	All year	All year	All year	All year	All year
Breeding life (years)	10–15	5–10	4	1–3	1	3	1	1	35
Breeding age (months)	54	9	10	6–7	2	3	2	2–3	180
Estrus cycle (days)	28	22	15–28	15–16	4–5	16–19	4	4–5	27–28
Duration of estrus (days)	1–6	7–13	4–19	30	1	1	16	1	2–8
Gestation period (days)	164	63	63	31	20	67	16	21	267
Litter size (number)	1	3–6	1–6	1–13	1–12	1–5	1–12	6–9	1
Birth weight (grams)	500–700	1100–2200	125	100	1.5	75–100	2.0	5.6	
Opening of eyes (days)	At birth	8–12	8–12	10	11	At birth	15	11	At birth
Weaning age (weeks)	16–24	6	6–9	18	3	2	3–4	3–4	
Weight at weaning (grams)	4400	5800	3000	1000–	11–12	250	35	10–12	

Note: Data obtained from various sources including: Ecobichon, D.J., *The Basis of Toxicity Testing*, CRC Press, Inc., Boca Raton, FL, 1992,[1] Chap. 2, Table 1; Spector, S., *Handbook of Biological Data*, W.B. Saunders Company, Philadelphia, PA, 1956,[2] various tables; Altman, P.L. and Dittmer, D.S., *Biology Data Book*, 2nd ed., Vol. I, Federation of American Societies for Experimental Biology, 1972,[3] various tables.

[a] Monkey = *Macaca mulatta*.

Table 79   Species Variability in Parameters Involving Spermatogenesis

Parameter	Mouse	Rat	Hamster	Rabbit	Dog	Monkey	Human
Spermatogenesis duration (days)	26–35	48–53	35	28–40			74
Duration of cycle of seminiferous epithelium (days)	8.6	12.9		10.7	13.6	9.5	16
Life span of:							
B-type spermatogonia (days)	1.5	2.0		1.3	4.0	2.9	6.3
L + Z spermatocytes (days)	4.7	7.8		7.3	5.2	6.0	9.3
P + D spermatocytes (days)	8.3	12.2		10.7	13.5	9.5	15.6
Golgi spermatids (days)	1.7	2.9		2.1	6.9	1.8	7.9
Cap spermatids (days)	3.5	5.0		5.2	3.0	3.7	1.6
Testis weight (grams)	0.2	3.7	1.8	6.4	12.0	4.9	34.0
Daily sperm production							
per gram testis (× 10^6)	54	14–22	22	25	20	23	4.4
per individual (× 10^6)	5–6	80–90	70	160	300	1100	125
Sperm reserve in cauda at sexual rest (× 10^6)	49	440	575	1600		5700	420
Sperm storage in epididymal tissue (× 10^6)							
Caput	20		200				
Corpus	7	300	175				420
Cauda	40–50	400	200				
Transit time through epidymis at sexual rest (days)							
Caput and corpus	3.1	3.0		3.0	?	4.9	1.8
Cauda	5.6	5.1		9.7	?	5.6	3.7
Ejaculate volume (ml)	0.04	0.2	0.1	1.0	?	?	3.0
Ejaculated sperm (10^6/ml)	5.0	?	?	150	?	?	80.0
Sperm transit time from vagina to tube	15–60 min	30–60 min		3–4 hr	20 min		15–30 min

Source: Data obtained from various sources, including: Altman, P.L. and Dittmer, D.S., (1972)[3]; Eddy, E.M. and O'Brien, D.A. (1989)[4]; Blazak, W.F. (1989)[5]; Zenick, H. and Clegg, E.D. (1989)[6]; and Spector, W.S. Ed. (1956).[2]

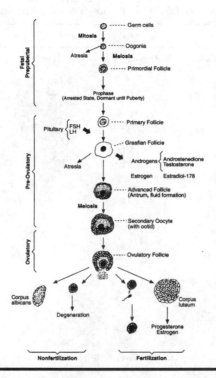

Figure 3   A general scheme of mammalian oogenesis, showing the fetal-prepu-
bertal development of the primordial follicles that lie in an arrested state until
puberty, at which time primary follicles begin to develop in response to pre-
ovulatory levels of pituitary follicle-stimulating hormone (FSH) and luteinizing
hormone (LH), with the formation of the Graffian follicle and, subsequently, the
advanced follicle which undergoes meiosis to produce a haploid oocyte. At the
ovulatory stage, one mature ovum is released form each follicle. If the ovum is
fertilized, the follicle becomes a steroid-secreting body, the corpus luteum,
essential for the maintenance of the pregnancy. If fertilization does not occur,
the follicle degenerates into a mass of cells, the corpus albicans. (From Ecobichon, D.J., *The Basis of Toxicity Testing*, CRC Press, Boca Raton, FL, 1992, chap.
5, Fig. 4.)[1]

Table 80 Species Variability in Parameters Involving Oogenesis

Parameter	Mouse	Rat	Guinea Pig	Hamster	Rabbit	Cat	Dog	Monkey	Human
Sexual maturity (days)	28	46–53	84	42–54	120–240	210–245	270–425	1642	
Duration of estrus (days)	9–20 hr	9–20 hr	6–11 hr		30	4	9	4–6	2–8
Ovulation time (days)	2–3 hr	9–20 hr	10 hr		10 hr	24–56 hr	1–3	9–20	15
Ovulation type[a]	S	S	S	S	I	I	S	S	S
No. ova released	8	10	?	7	10	4–6	8–10	1	1
Follicle size (mm)	0.5	0.9	0.8		1.8		10		
Ovum diameter (mm)	0.07–0.087	0.07–0.076	0.075–0.107		0.110–0.146	0.12–0.13	0.135–0.145	0.109–0.173	0.089–0.091
Zona pellucida (mm membrane thickness)			0.012		0.011–0.023	0.012–0.115	0.135	0.012–0.034	0.019–0.035
Transport time (to reach site of implantation) (days)	4.5	3.0	3.5	3.0	2.5–4	4–8	6–8	3.0	3.0
Implantation (days)	4.5–5.0	5.5–6.0	6.0	4.5–5.0	7–8	13–14	13–14	9–11	8–13
Rate of transport of sperm to oviduct (min)	15	15–30	15		5–10				5–60
Rate of transport of embryo to uterus (hr)	72	95–100	80–85		50				80
Fertile life of spermatozoa in female tract (hr)	6	14	21–22		30–32				24–48
Rate of transport of ova in female tract (hr)	8–12	12–14	20	5–12	6–8				24
Segmentation (to form blastocele) (days)	2.5–4.0	4.5	5–6	3.25	3–4				5–8
Primitive streak (days)	7.0	8.5	10.0	6.0	6.5	13.0	13.0	18.0	
Duration of organogenesis (days)	7.5–16	9–17	11–25	7–14	7–20	14–26	14–30	20–45	
Gestational length (days)	20–21	21–22	65–68	16–17	31–32	58–71	57–66	164–168	

[a] Ovulation type: I, induced; S, spontaneous.

Source. Data obtained from various sources, including: Ecobichon, D.J. (1992)[1]; Spector, S. (1956)[2]; Altman, P... and Dittmer, D.S. (1972)[3]; Eddy, E.M. and O'Brien, D.A. (1989)[4]; Manson, J.M., and Kang, Y.J. (1989).[7]

Table 81   Fertility and Reproductive Indices Used in Single and Multigeneration Studies

Index	Derivation
Mating	$= \dfrac{\text{No. confirmed copulations}}{\text{No. of estrous cycles required}} \times 100$
Male fertility	$= \dfrac{\text{No. males impregnating females}}{\text{No. males exposed to fertile, nonpregnant females}} \times 100$
Female fertility	$= \dfrac{\text{No. of females confirmed pregnant}}{\text{No. of females housed with fertile male}} \times 100$
Female fecundity	$= \dfrac{\text{No. of females confirmed pregnant}}{\text{No. of confirmed copulations}} \times 100$
Implantation	$= \dfrac{\text{No. of implantations}}{\text{No. of pregnant females}} \times 100$
Preimplantation loss	$= \dfrac{\text{Corpora lutea} - \text{No. of implants}}{\text{No. of Corpora lutea}} \times 100$
Parturition incidence	$= \dfrac{\text{No. of females giving birth}}{\text{No. of females confirmed pregnant}} \times 100$
Live litter size	$= \dfrac{\text{No. of litters with live pups}}{\text{No. of females confirmed pregnant}} \times 100$
Live birth	$= \dfrac{\text{No. viable pups born/litter}}{\text{No. pups born/litter}} \times 100$
Viability	$= \dfrac{\text{No. of viable pups born}}{\text{No. of dead pups born}} \times 100$
Survival	$= \dfrac{\text{No. of pups viable on day 1}}{\text{No. of viable pups born}} \times 100$
Pup death (day 1–4)	$= \dfrac{\text{No. of pups dying, postnatal days 1–4}}{\text{No. of viable pups born}} \times 100$
Pup death (days 5–21)	$= \dfrac{\text{No. of pups dying, postnatal days 5–21}}{\text{No. of viable pups born}} \times 100$

Table 81   Fertility and Reproductive Indices Used in Single and Multigeneration Studies (Continued)

Index	Derivation
Sex ratio (at birth)	$= \dfrac{\text{No. of male offspring}}{\text{No. of female offspring}} \times 100$
Sex ratio (day 4) (day 21)	$= \dfrac{\text{No. of male offspring}}{\text{No. of female offspring}} \times 100$

Source. From Ecobichon, D.J. (1992)[1]

Table 82   Basic Developmental Toxicity Testing Protocol

Phase	Time	Developmental Toxicity Testing[a]
Acclimation period	Variable number of weeks	No exposure of the animals to the test agent
Cohabitation period	Day of mating determined (Day 0)	No exposure of the animals to the test agent
Pre-embryonic period	Day of mating through Day 5,[b] 6,[c] 7[d] of pregnancy	
Period of major embryonic organogenesis	Day 5, 6, or 7 through Day 15[b,c] or 18[d] of pregnancy	Groups of pregnant animals exposed to the test agent
Fetal period	Day 15 or 18 through Day 18,[b] 21,[c] or 30[d] of pregnancy	No exposure of the pregnant animals to the test agent
Term	Day 18,[b] 22,[c] or 31[d] of pregnancy	Females sacrificed (to preclude cannibalization of malformed fetuses), cesarean section performed, and young examined externally and internally

[a] Usually a sham-treated control group and three agent-treated groups are used with 20 to 25 mice or rats and 15 to 18 rabbits per group. The dose levels are chosen with the goal of no maternal or developmental effects in the low-dose group and at least maternal toxicity in the high-dose group (failure to gain or loss of weight during dosing, reduced feed and/or water consumption, increased clinical signs, or no more than 10% maternal death).

[b] Mice.

[c] Rats.

[d] Rabbits.

Source: Adapted from Johnson, E.M. (1990).[8]

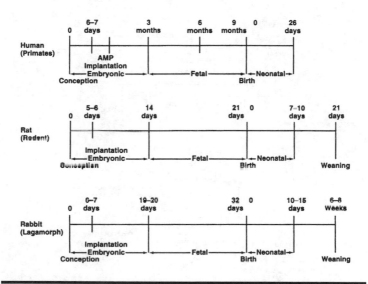

Figure 4   Developmental stages and timelines in the human, rat, and rabbit. AMP: Anticipated menstrual period. Average human menstrual cycle is 28 days, with ovulation occurring about 14 days. Rabbit ovulates following coitus. (Adapted from Miller, R.K., Kellogg, C.K., and Saltzman, R.A., 1987, chap. 7.)[9]

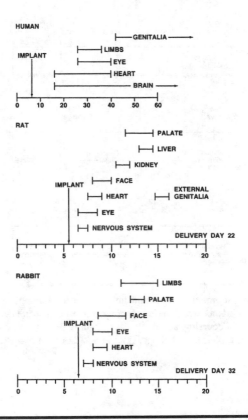

Figure 5   Critical periods of embryogenesis in the human, rat, and rabbit (days of gestation). When the emphasis is on the appearance of birth defects rather than general developmental toxicity, be aware of the extremely short duration of the "target-windows" in the animal surrogates. To produce birth defects rather than general developmental toxicity may require a concentration of the test agent which would kill the dam or destroy the pregnancy if delivered more than the one or two days included in the "target interval." (Adapted from Ecobichon, D.J. 1992, chap. 5.)[1]

References

1. Ecobichon, D.J., Reproductive toxicology, in *The Basis of Toxicity Testing*, CRC Press, Boca Raton, FL, 1992, chap. 5, p. 83-112.

2. Spector, W.S., Ed., *Handbook of Biological Data*, W.B. Saunders, Philadelphia, 1956.

3. Altman, P.L. and Dittmer, D.S., *Biology Data Book*, 2nd ed., Vol. 1, Federation of American Societies for Experimental Biology, Bethesda, MD, 1972.

4. Eddy, E.M. and O'Brien, D.A., Biology of the gamete: maturation, transport, and fertilization, in *Toxicology of the Male and Female Reproductive Systems*, Working, P.K., Ed., Hemisphere, Washington, D.C., 1989, chap. 3, p. 31-100.

5. Blazak, W.F., Significance of cellular endpoints in assessment of male reproductive toxicity, in *Toxicology of the Male and Female Reproductive Systems*, Working, P.K., Ed., Hemisphere Washington, D.C., 1989, chap. 6, p. 157-172.

6. Zenick, H. and Clegg, E.D., Assessment of male reproductive toxicity: a risk assessment approach, in *Principles and Methods of Toxicology*, Hayes, A.W., Ed., Raven Press, New York, 1989, chap. 10, p. 275-309.

7. Manson, J.M. and Kang, Y.S., Test methods for assessing female reproductive and developmental toxicology, in *Principles and Methods of Toxicology*, 2nd ed., Hayes, A.W., Ed., Raven Press, New York, 1989, chap. 11, p. 311-359.

8. Johnson, E.M., The effects of riboviron on development and reproduction: a critical review of published and unpublished studies in experimental animals, *J. Am. Coll. Toxicol.*, 9, 551, 1990.

9. Miller, R.K., Kellogg, C.K., and Saltzman, R.A., Reproductive and perinatal toxicology, in *Handbook of Toxicology*, Haley, T.J. and Berndt, W.O., Eds., Hemisphere Publishing, Washington, D.C., 1987, chap. 7.

Section 10:
Clinical Pathology

Table 83   Approximate Blood Volumes in Animals Typically Used in Nonclinical Toxicology Research

Species	Typical Body Weight (kg)	Total Volume (ml)	Weekly Sampling	Monthly Sampling	At Necropsy
Mouse	0.03	2	0.075	0.2	1
Rat	0.3	20	1	2	10
Dog	12.0	1000	50	100	400
Monkey[a]	3.0	200	10	20	100
Rabbit	3.0	200	10	20	100

Blood Volume (ml) column heading spans Total Volume, Weekly Sampling, Monthly Sampling, At Necropsy.

[a]   Rhesus or cynomolgus.

Source: Adapted from Loeb, W.F. and Quimby, F.W. (1989).[1]

Table 84   Mean Control Ranges of Typical Serum Clinical Chemistry Measurements in CD® Rats

Parameter	10–12 Weeks Old	18–20 Weeks Old	32–34 Weeks Old	58–60 Weeks Old	84–86 Weeks Old	108–110 Weeks Old
Alanine aminotransferase (ALT) (IU/l)	10–40	10–50	10–50	20–60	20–60	20–60
Albumin (g/dl)	3.4–4.1 (M) 3.5–4.5 (F)	3.3–4.2 (M) 3.5–4.7 (F)	3.5–4.0 (M) 4.0–5.0 (F)	3.0–3.8 (M) 3.5–4.5 (F)	3.0–4.0 (M) 3.7–4.5 (F)	2.7–3.5 (M) 3.3–3.7 (F)
Albumin/globulin ratio	1.0–1.5	1.0–1.5	1.0–1.5	0.75–1.75	0.75–1.75	0.75–1.5
Alkaline phosphatase (IU/l)	140–300 (M) 80–100 (F)	50–150 (M) 25–150 (F)	50–150 (M) 25–100 (F)	50–150 (M) 25–100 (F)	50–150 (M) 25–100 (F)	50–100 (M) 25–100 (F)
Aspartate aminotransferase (AST) (IU/l)	45–90	45–100	45–120	60–120	75–150	75–150
Bile acids, total (µmol/l)	20–60	20–60	—[a]	—	—	—
Bilirubin, total (mg/dl)	0.2–0.4	0.1–0.5	0.1–0.5	0.1–0.5	0.1–0.5	0.1–0.4
Calcium (mg/dl)	9.8–12.0	9.8–12.0	9.8–12.0	9.8–12.0	9.8–12.0	9.8–12.0
Chloride (mEq/l)	97–105	97–105	95–105	97–105	97–105	97–105
Cholesterol, total (mg/dl)	50–85	50–100	70–140	60–150	130–180 (M) 100–150 (F)	130–180 (M) 90–150 (F)
Creatine kinase (CK) (IU/l)	50–400	50–300	50–500	—	—	—
Creatinine (mg/dl)	0.3–0.8	0.3–0.9	0.3–1.0	0.4–0.8	0.4–0.8	0.4–1.3
gamma-Glutamyltransferase (γGT) (IU/l)	0–2	0–2	0–3	0–5	0–7	0–5
Globulin (g/dl)	2.5–4.0	2.5–4.0	2.0–4.5	2.0–4.5	2.0–4.5	2.0–4.5
Glucose (mg/dl)	90–175	100–175	100–200	100–200	100–175	100–175
Lactate dehydrogenase (LDH) (IU/l)	50–400	50–400	50–500	—	—	—
Phosphorus, inorganic (mg/dl)	7.0–10.0	4.0–8.5	4.0–8.0	3.5–7.0	3.5–8.0	4.0–7.0

Potassium (mEq/l)	5.5–8.0	4.0–7.0	4.0–7.0	4.0–7.0	3.5–6.0	3.5–6.0
Protein, total (g/dl)	6.2–7.6 (M) 6.3–8.2 (F)	6.2–7.8 (M) 6.5–8.5 (F)	6.2–8.0 (M) 7.0–9.0 (F)	6.0–8.0 (M) 6.5–8.5 (F)	6.3–7.6 (M) 5.7–8.0 (F)	5.7–6.5 (M) 6.3–7.1 (F)
Sodium (mEq/l)	140–153	140–153	140–153	140–153	140–153	140–145
Sorbitol dehydrogenase (SDH) (IU/l)	10–30	10–30	10–30	—	—	—
Triglycerides (mg/dl)	50–125	50–200	50–200	50–300	75–400	50–300
Urea nitrogen (BUN) (mg/dl)	12–18	12–20	12–20	12–18	12–18	12–30

[a] — = data unavailable.

Source: Adapted from Levine, B.S. (1979–1993)[2] and Charles River Laboratories (1993).[3]

Table 85   Mean Control Ranges of Typical Serum Clinical Chemistry Measurements in F-344 Rats

Parameter	12–14 Weeks Old	18–20 Weeks Old	32–34 Weeks Old	58–60 Weeks Old	84–86 Weeks Old	110–112 Weeks Old
Alanine aminotransferase (ALT) (IU/l)	25–45	30–62	20–40	56–100 (M) 33–65 (F)	41–80 (M) 32–50 (F)	25–60
Albumin (g/dl)	3.8–4.7	3.0–5.0	4.0–5.0	3.8–5.0	3.8–5.0	3.5–5.0
Albumin/globulin ratio	1.5–2.3	1.1–2.5	1.5–2.0	1.4–1.9	1.4–2.0	1.2–1.8
Alkaline phosphatase (IU/l)	200–300 (M) 150–250 (F)	58–154 (M) 45–120 (F)	45–80	31–68	—[a]	—
Aspartate aminotransferase (AST) (IU/l)	50–90	50–100	—	—	—	—
Bile acids, total (μmol/l)	10–50	—	—	—	—	—
Bilirubin, total (mg/dl)	—	0.1–0.5	0.1–0.4	0.1–0.5	0.1–0.5	0.1–0.4
Calcium (mg/dl)	—	9.5–12.0	9.5–11.2	9.5–11.5	9.5–11.5	9.8–11.7
Chloride (mEq/l)	—	97–115	98–110	100–112	97–100	104–113
Cholesterol, total (mg/dl)	70–100 (M) 90–135 (F)	50–80 (M) 80–120 (F)	50–80 (M) 85–130 (F)	68–125 (M) 110–150 (F)	100–120	125–175
Creatine kinase (CK) (IU/l)	60–300	100–400	300–700	300–500	100–500	100–400
Creatine (mg/dl)	0.5–1.0	0.4–0.8	—	—	—	—
Globulin (g/dl)	1.5–2.5	1.2–2.8	2.0–3.0	2.3–3.5	2.0–3.0	2.2–3.2
Glucose (mg/dl)	100–180	90–170	80–130	90–140	90–140	90–140
Lactate dehydrogenase (LDH) (IU/l)	—	500–800	400–800	150–400	—	—
Phosphorus, inorganic (mg/dl)	—	3.9–7.3	—	—	—	—
Potassium (mEq/l)	—	3.6–5.9	4.0–5.7	4.1–5.5	4.0–5.2	4.0–5.1

Protein, total (g/dl)	6.0–7.2	5.7–7.6	6.2–7.5	6.5–7.6	6.0–7.8	6.1–8.0
Sodium (mEq/l)	—	140–155	142–158	142–156	138–149	138–146
Sorbitol dehydrogenase (SDH) (IU/l)	15–60	5–25	5–35	—	—	—
Triglycerides (mg/dl)	100–400 (M) 25–130 (F)	75–150 (M) 35–70 (F)	125–190 (M) 30–70 (F)	90–175 (M) 40–85 (F)	110–240 (M) 60–145 (F)	80–220
Urea nitrogen (BUN) (mg/dl)	15–25	10–26	12–24	10–20	10–20	12–25

[a] — = data unavailable.

Source: Adapted from Levine, B.S. (1979–1993)[2]; NIEHS (1985)[4]; and Burns, K.F., Timmons, E.H., and Poiley, S.M. (1971).[5]

Table 86   Mean Control Ranges of Typical Serum Clinical Chemistry Measurements in B6C3F$_1$ Mice

Parameter	12–14 Weeks Old	18–20 Weeks Old	32–34 Weeks Old	58–60 Weeks Old	84–86 Weeks Old	110–112 Weeks Old
Alanine aminotransferase (ALT) (IU/l)	20–50	25–100	22–90	20–50	23–60	20–60
Albumin (g/dl)	2.3–4.4	2.5–4.2	2.7–3.8	3.0–4.0	3.0–3.9	3.0–4.1
Albumin/globulin ratio	1.0–2.0	0.8–2.0	1.2–1.9	1.3–1.9	1.3–2.0	1.3–2.0
Alkaline phosphatase (IU/l)	30–80 (M)	20–55 (M)	—[a]	—	—	—
	40–140 (F)	45–85 (F)				
Aspartate aminotransferase (AST) (IU/l)	40–100	64–180	—	—	—	—
Bilirubin, total (mg/dl)	—	0.1–0.5	0.1–0.5	0.1–0.5	0.1–0.5	0.1–0.5
Calcium (mg/dl)	—	8.2–11.8	—	—	—	—
Chloride (mEq/l)	—	110–128	—	—	—	—
Cholesterol, total (mg/dl)	90–160	80–130	85–150	80–150	90–160	90–175
Creatine kinase (CK) (IU/l)	50–300	—	—	—	—	—
Creatinine (mg/dl)	0.3–0.8	0.2–0.8	—	—	—	—
Globulin (g/dl)	1.5–2.5	1.0–2.7	1.6–2.4	1.8–3.1	1.6–3.0	1.8–3.0
Glucose (mg/dl)	125–200	81–165	115–170	115–170	115–170	115–170
Phosphorus, inorganic (mg/dl)	—	—	—	—	—	—
Potassium (mEq/l)	—	3.6–7.3	—	—	—	—
Protein, total (g/dl)	4.5–5.5	4.0–6.0	4.2–6.2	4.8–6.5	4.8–6.6	5.4–6.5
Sodium (mEq/l)	—	147–163	—	—	—	—
Sorbitol dehydrogenase (SDH) (IU/l)	15–50	18–57	—	—	—	—
Triglycerides (mg/dl)	75–175	75–130	100–173	90–190	110–160	90–175
Urea nitrogen (BUN) (mg/dl)	15–35	12–34	12–27	12–24	10–24	15–28

[a] — = data unavailable.
Source: Adapted from Levine, B.S. (1979–1993)[2] and NIEHS (1985).[4]

Table 87 Mean Control Ranges of Typical Serum Clinical Chemistry Measurements in CD-1 and BALB/c Mice

Parameter	<1-Year-Old CD-1	>1-Year-Old CD-1	1–3-Month-Old BALB/c	6–12-Month-Old BALB/c
Alanine aminotransferase (ALT) (IU/l)	30–250 (M) 30–100 (F)	20–200 (M) 20–80 (F)	—[a] —	— —
Albumin (g/dl)	—	—	1.6–2.6	1.3–2.6
Albumin/globulin ratio	—	—	—	—
Alkaline phosphatase (IU/l)	30–70	20–75	75–275	47–102
Aspartate aminotransferase (AST) (IU/l)	75–300	75–200	40–140	70–110
Bilirubin, total (mg/dl)	0.2–0.8	0.2–0.8	0.5–1.2	0.4–1.0
Calcium (mg/dl)	8.5–11.5	6.7–11.5	7.8–10.8	6.5–9.6
Chloride (mEq/l)	110–125	110–135	—	—
Cholesterol, total (mg/dl)	90–170 (M) 60–125 (F)	60–170 (M) 50–100 (F)	165–295	100–300
Creatine kinase (CK) (IU/l)	—	—	—	—
Creatinine (mg/dl)	0.3–1.0	0.2–2.0	—	—
Globulin (g/dl)	—	—	—	—
Glucose (mg/dl)	75–175	60–150	75–150	40–160
Phosphorus, inorganic (mg/dl)	7.5–11.0	6.0–10.0	4.5–8.9	4.7–7.2
Potassium (mEq/1)	6.5–9.0	6.6–9.0	—	—
Protein, total (g/dl)	4.5–6.0	3.5–5.6	4.4–6.0	4.4–6.4
Sodium (mEq/1)	145–160	155–170	—	—
Triglycerides (mg/dl)	60–140 (M) 50–100 (F)	40–150 (M) 25–75 (F)	— —	— —
Urea nitrogen (BUN) (mg/dl)	20–40	20–70	10–30	10–30

[a] — = data unavailable.

Source: Adapted from Frith, C.H., Suber, R.L., and Umholtz, R. (1980)[6] and Wolford, S.T., Schroer, R.A., Gohs, F.X., Gallo, P.P., Brodeck, M., Falk, H.B., and Ruhren, R.J. (1986).[7]

Table 88 Mean Control Ranges of Typical Serum Clinical Chemistry Measurements in Beagle Dogs

Parameter	6–8 Months Old	9–11 Months Old	12–14 Months Old	15–18 Months Old	19–30 Months Old
Alanine aminotransferase (ALT) (IU/l)	20–40	20–40	20–40	20–40	20–40
Albumin (g/dl)	2.5–3.5	2.5–3.5	2.5–3.5	2.5–4.0	2.7–4.5
Albumin/globulin ratio	0.8–1.5	0.8–1.5	0.8–1.5	0.8–2.0	0.8–2.0
Alkaline phosphatase (IU/l)	120–160 (M) 100–130 (F)	70–120 (M) 60–100 (F)	50–100	35–100	35–100
Aspartate aminotransferase (AST) (IU/l)	30–45	30–50	25–50	25–50	25–50
Bilirubin, total (mg/dl)	0.1–0.7	0.1–0.7	0.1–0.7	0.1–0.3	0.1–0.3
Calcium (mg/dl)	9.0–11.5	9.0–11.5	9.0–11.5	10.0–11.3	10.0–11.5
Chloride (mEq/l)	100–115	100–115	100–115	105–119	105–115
Cholesterol, total (mg/dl)	150–250	125–250	125–250	125–250	125–225
Creatine kinase (CK) (IU/l)	100–400	100–400	100–400	—[a]	—
Creatinine (mg/dl)	0.5–0.8	0.7–0.9	0.7–0.9	—	—
gamma-Glutamyltransferase (γGT) (IU/l)	0–5	0–5	0–5	—	—
Globulin (g/dl)	2.5–3.5	2.5–3.5	2.5–3.5	2.5–3.5	2.5–3.5
Glucose (mg/dl)	100–130	100–130	100–130	70–110	70–110
Haptoglobin (mg/dl)	50–200	50–150	25–100	—	—
Lactate dehydrogenase (LDH) (IU/l)	30–100	30–100	30–100	—	—

Phosphorus, inorganic (mg/dl)	6.0–9.0	4.0–6.0	3.0–5.0	3.0–5.0	3.0–4.7
Potassium (mEq/l)	4.2–5.0	4.2–5.0	4.2–5.0	4.1–5.1	4.2–5.2
Protein, total (g/dl)	5.5–6.5	5.5–6.5	5.5–6.5	5.5–6.5	5.7–6.6
Sodium (mEq/l)	143–147	143–147	143–147	143–153	143–153
Triglycerides (mg/dl)	30–60	30–75	30–75	—	—
Urea nitrogen (BUN) (mg/dl)	10–20	10–20	10–20	10–20	10–20

[a] — = data unavailable.

Source: Adapted from Levine, B.S. (1979–1993)[2]; Clarke, D. Tupari, G., Walker, R., and Smith, G. (1992)[6]; and Pickrell, J.A., Schluter, S.J., Belasich, J.J., Stewart, E.V., Meyer, J., Hubbs, C.H., and Jones, R.K. (1974)[9]; Kaspar, L.V. and Norris, W.P. (1977)[10].

Table 89   Mean Control Ranges of Typical Serum Clinical Chemistry Measurements in Nonhuman Primates

Parameter	3–7-Year-Old Cynomolgus	1–2-Year-Old Rhesus	3–7-Year-Old Rhesus	<1.5-Year-Old Marmoset	>1.5-Year-Old Marmoset	1–5-Year-Old Baboon	6–15-Year-Old Baboon
Alanine amino-transferase (ALT) (IU/l)	20–60	20–50	15–40	45–75	40–70	15–50	20–50
Albumin (g/dl)	3.5–4.8	3.0–4.5	3.2–4.5	3.5–5.8	3.5–5.8	3.1–4.5	2.0–4.5
Albumin/globulin ratio	1.0–1.5	1.0–1.5	1.0–1.5	1.0–1.5	1.0–1.5	1.0–1.5	1.0–1.5
Alkaline phosphatase (IU/l)	300–800 (M) 200–500 (F)	200–600	70–300	100–250	35–80	200–1000	100–200
Amylase (IU/l)	200–500	—ᵃ	—	1000–2000	500–1500	200–400	200–500
Aspartate amino-transferase (AST) (IU/l)	25–60	25–60	15–70	100–200	100–200	18–35	20–35
Bilirubin, total (mg/dl)	0.3–0.8	0.1–0.8	0.1–0.6	0.1–0.9	0.1–0.9	0.3–0.7	0.3–0.5
Calcium (mg/dl)	9.0–11.0	8.2–10.5	8.5–10.3	8.1–12.4	8.5–11.7	8.0–9.5	7.5–10.0
Chloride (mEq/l)	100–115	103–115	97–110	80–110	93–119	105–115	100–110
Cholesterol, total (mg/dl)	90–160	90–160	90–170	90–210	105–230	75–200	70–125
Creatine kinase (CK) (IU/l)	140–200	200–1000	200–600	—	—	—	—
Creatinine (mg/dl)	0.7–1.2	0.5–0.9	0.7–1.2	0.2–1.0	0.2–1.0	0.8–1.2	1.0–1.8
gamma-Glutamyl-transferase (γGT) (IU/l)	40–90	—	10–60	—	—	—	—
Globulin (g/dl)	3.0–4.5	3.0–4.0	3.0–4.0	2.5–4.0	3.5–4.0	2.5–4.0	2.5–4.5

Glucose (mg/dl)	50–100	50–100	41–80	180–275	130–240	50–125	50–140
Lactate dehydrogenase (LDH) (IU/l)	300–600	130–600	125–600	125–500	100–350	100–400	100–350
Phosphorus, inorganic (mg/dl)	4.0–7.0	3.2–5.0	3.0–5.3	5.5–9.8	4.0–7.5	4.7–7.5	1.3–4.5
Potassium (mEq/l)	3.0–4.5	3.0–4.2	3.1–4.1	3.5–5.0	3.0–4.8	3.2–4.3	3.7–4.8
Protein, total (g/dl)	7.0–9.0	6.7–8.0	7.0–8.3	5.5–7.5	6.0–8.0	6.0–8.0	6.0–7.5
Sodium (mEq/l)	140–153	144–150	142–148	150–170	150–170	142–158	142–158
Triglycerides (mg/dl)	30–70	50–200	50–200	75–200	75–200	25–60	30–125
Urea nitrogen (BUN) (mg/dl)	15–25	14–26	14–25	17–35	15–32	10–25	10–25

[a] — = data unavailable.

Source: Adapted from Levine, B.S. (1979–1993)[2]; Clarke, D., Tupari, G., Walker, R., and Smith, G. (1992)[8]; Kapeghian, L.C., and Verlangieri, A.J. (1984)[11]; Davy, C.W., Jackson, M.R., and Walker, S. (1984)[12]; Yarbrough. L.W., ˉollett, J.L., Montrey, R.D., and Beattie, R.J. (1984)[13]; and Hack, C.A., and Gleiser, C.A. (1982).[14]

Table 90   Mean Control Ranges of Typical Serum Clinical Chemistry Measurements in New Zealand White Rabbits

Parameter	15–20 Weeks Old	25–40 Weeks Old	1–2 Years Old
Alanine aminotransferase (ALT) (IU/l)	25–70	25–70	25–70
Albumin (g/dl)	3.8–5.0	3.5–4.7	3.0–4.5
Albumin/globulin ratio	2.0–3.0	2.0–3.0	2.0–3.0
Alkaline phosphatase (IU/l)	50–120	40–120	15–90
Aspartate aminotransferase (AST) (IU/l)	20–50	10–35	10–30
Bilirubin, total (mg/dl)	0.1–0.5	0.1–0.5	0.2–0.6
Calcium (mg/dl)	12.0–14.0	11.0–14.0	12.0–15.0
Chloride (mEq/l)	97–110	96–108	100–110
Cholesterol, total (mg/dl)	20–60	20–60	20–60
Creatine kinase (CK) (IU/l)	200–800	200–1000	200–1000
Creatinine (mg/dl)	1.0–1.6	0.8–1.6	0.8–1.7
gamma-Glutamyltransferase (γGT) (IU/l)	—[a]	0–10	0–6
Globulin (g/dl)	1.4–1.9	1.5–2.2	1.5–2.5
Glucose (mg/dl)	100–160	100–175	80–140
Lactate dehydrogenase (LDH) (IU/l)	50–200	50–200	35–125
Phosphorus, inorganic (mg/dl)	4.6–7.2	4.0–7.0	3.0–5.0
Potassium (mEq/l)	4.0–5.2	4.0–5.0	3.3–4.5
Protein, total (g/dl)	5.4–6.6	5.5–7.0	5.5–7.5
Sodium (mEq/l)	132–144	132–145	132–150
Urea nitrogen (BUN) (mg/dl)	10–20	12–22	12–25

[a] — = data unavailable.

Source: Adapted from Levine, B.S. (1979–1993)[2]; Hewett, C.D., Innes, D.J., Savory, J., and Wills, M.R. (1989)[15]; and Yu, L., Pragay, D.A., Chang, D., and Wicher, K. (1979).[16]

Table 91   Mean Control Ranges of Typical Hematology Measurements in CD® Rats

Parameters	10–12 Weeks Old	18–20 Weeks Old	32–34 Weeks Old	58–60 Weeks Old	84–86 Weeks Old	108–110 Weeks Old
Activated partial thromboplastin time (sec)	14.0–20.0 (M) 12.0–18.0 (F)	14.0–20.0 (M) 13.0–18.0 (F)	14.0–17.0 (M) 13.0–16.0 (F)	16.0–19.0 (M) 15.0–18.0 (F)	—[a]	—
Erythrocyte count (10^6/mm^3)	6.8–8.5 (M) 7.0–8.2 (F)	7.0–9.8 (M) 6.5–9.2 (F)	7.0–9.6 (M) 6.5–8.8 (F)	7.0–9.2 (M) 6.5–8.5 (F)	7.0–9.2 (M) 6.0–8.5 (F)	6.2–8.2 (M) 5.8–8.0 (F)
Fibrinogen (mg/dl)	—	200–300 (M) 130–190 (F)	—	—	—	—
Hematocrit (%)	40.0–48.0	36.0–52.0	36.0–50.0	38.0–48.0	38.0–50.0	35.0–45.0
Hemoglobin (g/dl)	14.0–17.0	14.0–17.0	14.0–17.0	14.0–17.0	14.0–17.0	12.0–15.0
Leukocyte count, total (10^3/mm^3)	6.0–18.0 (M) 4.0–14.0 (F)	6.0–19.0 (M) 5.0–14.0 (F)	6.0–18.0 (M) 4.0–11.0 (F)	5.0–15.0 (M) 3.0–9.0 (F)	10.0–15.0 (M) 6.0–10.0 (F)	5.0–18.0 (M) 3.0–12.0 (F)
Mean corpuscular hemoglobin (pg)	19.0–22.0	16.0–20.0	17.0–21.0	16.0–21.0	16.0–20.0	16.0–20.0
Mean corpuscular hemoglobin conc. (g/dl)	33.0–38.0	31.0–38.0	31.0–38.0	32.0–38.0	31.0–36.0	31.0–36.0
Mean corpuscular volume (fl)	53.0–63.0	50.0–60.0	45.0–60.0	46.0–58.0	48.0–56.0	50.0–63.0
Methemoglobin (% Hgb)	0.4–1.2	0.4–1.2	0.4–1.2	—	—	—
Platelet count (10^3/mm^3)	900–1300	800–1200	700–1200	700–1200	700–1200	700–1200
Prothrombin time (sec)	9.0–14.0	9.0–14.0	10.0–14.0	10.0–14.0	—	—
Reticulocyte count (% RBC)	0.2–1.0	0.2–0.8	0.2–0.8	—	—	—

[a] — = data not available.

Source: Adapted from Levine, B.S. (1979–1993)[2] and Charles River Laboratories (1993).[17]

Table 92   Mean Control Ranges of Typical Hematology Measurements in F-344 Rats

Parameters	10–12 Weeks Old	18–20 Weeks Old	32–34 Weeks Old	58–60 Weeks Old	84–86 Weeks Old	108–110 Weeks Old
Erythrocyte count (10^6/mm^3)	7.2–8.6	7.0–10.0	8.5–9.6	7.2–9.5	7.5–9.8	6.5–9.6
Hematocrit (%)	39.5–45.5	42.0–50.0	41.4–46.7	40.0–46.6	40.3–45.5	40.0–48.5
Hemoglobin (g/dl)	15.0–17.0	15.0–17.3	15.0–17.8	15.7–17.5	15.5–17.6	13.0–18.5
Leukocyte count, total (10^3/mm^3)	7.1–13.5 (M) 5.4–11.7 (F)	6.5–10.7 (M) 4.5–7.0 (F)	6.5–8.7 (M) 4.4–6.5 (F)	5.8–9.0 (M) 4.5–6.2 (F)	5.7–8.5 (M) 3.2–6.0 (F)	5.0–15.0 (M) 3.5–8.0 (F)
Mean corpuscular hemoglobin (pg)	18.5–21.0	17.5–20.8	18.5–21.0	18.1–20.7	18.0–20.5	18.5–22.0
Mean corpuscular hemoglobin conc. (g/dl)	36.6–39.6	35.3–39.2	37.8–40.0	36.9–40.5	37.0–40.6	36.3–40.9
Mean corpuscular volume (fl)	48.0–58.0	48.3–56.1	48.0–56.0	47.0–56.0	47.0–56.0	50.0–58.0
Methemoglobin (% Hgb)	—[a]	0–3.0	0–4.0	0–2.5	0–2.7	0–20
Platelet count (10^3/mm^3)	400–750	350–700	400–870	450–700	450–700	200–450
Reticulocyte count (% RBC)	1.0–2.0	0.7–2.0	0.8–2.0	0.8–2.0	0.3–1.5	0.5–2.5

[a] — = data not available.

Source: Adapted from Levine, B.S. (1979–1993)[2] and NIEHS (1985).[4]

Table 93 Mean Control Ranges of Typical Hematology Measurements in B6C3F$_1$ Mice

Parameters	12–14 Weeks Old	18–20 Weeks Old	32–34 Weeks Old	58–60 Weeks Old	84–86 Weeks Old	110–112 Weeks Old
Erythrocyte count (10^6/mm^3)	9.0–10.2	7.5–10.5	8.0–10.4	8.0–10.0	8.6–10.4	7.7–10.4
Hematocrit (%)	44.1–49.5	36.0–48.6	40.8–46.6	38.5–45.5	40.0–46.9	36.0–43.5
Hemoglobin (g/dl)	15.0–17.1	13.1–16.5	15.2–18.2	14.5–17.5	15.0–18.2	13.0–16.8
Leukocyte count, total (10^3/mm^3)	3.0–7.8 (M) 2.5–5.0 (F)	5.5–10.9 (M) 3.2–5.2 (F)	6.1–13.3 (M) 4.2–9.3 (F)	6.1–13.2 (M) 4.6–10.5 (F)	7.0–13.4 (M) 3.9–7.9 (F)	5.0–16.5 (M) 4.2–8.8 (F)
Mean corpuscular hemoglobin (pg)	16.6–18.8	16.9–20.2	16.4–18.9	15.8–18.0	15.9–18.3	15.7–18.7
Mean corpuscular hemoglobin conc. (g/dl)	34.6–38.4	34.6–40.4	37.1–41.2	36.5–39.0	36.2–19.4	35.7–38.8
Mean corpuscular volume (fl)	44.0–52.0	45.4–53.6	44.0–48.0	42.0–47.0	42.0–18.0	46.0–50.0
Methemoglobin (% Hgb)	—^{a}	0–3.0	0–2.5	0–1.5	0–0.9	0–1.0
Platelet count (10^3/mm^3)	700–1100	500–1000	800–1200	700–1200	400–1100	400–800
Reticulocyte count (% RBC)	0.5–2.0	1.0–3.9	0.4–2.8	0.4–1.6	0.2–2.3	0.5–2.5

^{a} — = data not available.

Source: Adapted from Levine, B.S. (1979–1993)[2] and NIEHS (1985).[4]

Table 94 Mean Control Ranges of Typical Hematology Measurements in CD-1 and BALB/c Mice

Parameters	1–3-Month-Old BALB/c	6–12-Month-Old BALB/c	<1-Year-Old CD-1	>1-Year-Old CD-1
Erythrocyte count (10^6/mm^3)	8.5–10.5	8.8–10.6	8.0–10.0	6.0–9.0
Hematocrit (%)	42.5–47.9	38.3–46.9	36.9–46.9	28.2–41.1
Hemoglobin (g/dl)	14.5–16.8	14.2–17.0	13.6–16.8	10.4–14.9
Leukocyte count, total (10^3/mm^3)	2.0–5.7	2.0–5.0	4.0–12.0 (M) 3.5–9.7 (F)	3.4–17.0 (M) 2.4–13.4 (F)
Mean corpuscular hemoglobin (pg)	15.8–18.4	15.1–17.5	16.1–18.6	15.1–18.4
Mean corpuscular hemoglobin conc. (g/dl)	34.2–38.1	35.1–40.6	34.8–38.2	34.6–37.6
Mean corpuscular volume (fl)	46.3–50.3	40.9–45.9	44.5–49.7	41.3–51.1
Platelet count (10^3/mm^3)	—[a]	—	700–1400	700–1500
Reticulocyte count (% RBC)	—	—	1.6–3.7	1.7–5.0

[a] — = data not available.

Modified from Frith et al. (1980)[6] and Wolford et al. (1986).[7]

Source: Adapted from Frith, C.H., Suber, R.L., and Umholtz, R. (1980)[6] and Wolford S.T., Schroer, R.A., Gohs, F.X., Gallo, P.P., Brodeck, M., Falk, H.B., and Ruhren, R.J. (1986).[7]

Table 95 Mean Control Ranges of Typical Hematology Measurements in Beagle Dogs

Parameters	6–8 Months Old	9–11 Months Old	12–14 Months Old	15–18 Months Old	19–30 Months Old
Activated partial thromboplastin time (sec)	9.0–13.0	9.0–13.0	9.0–13.0	9.0–13.0	9.0–13.0
Erythrocyte count (10^6/mm^3)	6.0–7.3	6.2–8.0	6.2–8.2	5.8–7.3	5.8–7.3
Fibrinogen (mg/dl)	150–300	100–200	—[a]	—	—
Hematocrit (%)	41.5–49.0	44.3–54.9	46.0–54.6	42.5–55.0	42.0–52.0
Hemoglobin (g/dl)	14.5–17.3	15.8–18.0	16.0–18.8	13.0–19.0	13.0–19.0
Leukocyte count, total (10^3/mm^3)	5.5–14.0	6.8–13.6	5.7–15.5	5.0–15.0	6.0–18.0
Mean corpuscular hemoglobin (pg)	21.5–25.1	21.6–24.9	22.0–25.2	22.5–26.0	23.0–26.0
Mean corpuscular hemoglobin conc. (g/dl)	33.0–37.0	33.0–36.4	34.0–36.0	30.0–34.0	30.0–34.0
Mean corpuscular volume (fl)	65.0–71.0	64.0–73.0	64.0–72.0	65.0–78.0	65.0–78.0
Methemoglobin (% Hgb)	0–2.0	0–1.5	0–1.5	—	—
Platelet count (10^3/mm^3)	150–400	150–400	150–400	150–400	150–400
Prothrombin time (sec)	6.2–8.4	6.8–8.4	6.2–8.8	6.5–9.0	6.5–9.0
Reticulocyte count (% RBC)	0–0.7	0–0.7	0–0.7	0–0.7	0–0.7

[a] — = data not available.

Source: Adapted from Levine, B.S. (1979–1993)[2], Bulgin, M.S., Munn, S.L., and Gee, S. (1970)[18]; and Jordan, J.E. (1977).[19]

Table 96 Mean Control Ranges of Typical Hematology Measurements in Nonhuman Primates

Parameter	3–7-Year-Old Cynomolgus	1–2-Year-Old Rhesus	3–7-Year-Old Rhesus	<1.5-Year-Old Marmoset	>1.5-Year-Old Marmoset	1–5-Year-Old Baboon	6–15-Year-Old Baboon
Activated partial thromboplastin time (sec)	15.5–22.7	15.0–22.0	15.0–22.0	—[a]	—	—	30–60
Erythrocyte count (10⁶/mm³)	4.5–7.2	4.4–5.8	4.2–6.2	4.2–6.2	4.6–6.8	4.2–5.7	4.0–5.3
Hematocrit (%)	31.5–37.9	31.5–39.2	29.3–39.0	30.0–42.1	37.7–47.5	31.0–43.0	34.0–42.0
Hemoglobin (g/dl)	10.4–12.4	10.8–13.5	9.8–13.1	12.6–15.0	13.5–16.8	10.8–13.5	10.3–13.1
Leukocyte count, total (10³/mm³)	5.3–13.4	4.5–13.3	4.3–12.2	5.5–13.0	4.6–11.3	4.9–13.0	4.8–13.9
Mean corpuscular hemoglobin (pg)	18.9–22.3	19.8–24.8	19.6–23.2	24.0–30.5	23.0–29.0	22.0–27.0	22.0–28.0
Mean corpuscular hemoglobin conc. (g/dl)	32.0–35.6	31.3–35.5	31.7–37.5	32.1–42.6	32.2–42.5	28.0–34.0	30.0–35.0
Mean corpuscular volume (fl)	57.1–63.9	66.0–74.0	56.0–70.0	66.0–76.0	68.0–77.0	63.0–80.00	75.0–91.0
Platelet count (10³/mm³)	150–400	200–600	200–500	200–500	200–500	200–500	200–500
Prothrombin time (sec)	11.5–14.0	9.9–12.2	11.2–14.4	—	—	—	9.0–13.0
Reticulocyte count (% RBC)	0–0.5	0–1.4	0–1.5	0–5.0	0–4.7	0–2.3	0–1.9

[a] — = data not available.

Source: Adapted from Levine, B.S. (1979–1993)[2]; Kapeghian, L.C., and Verlangieri, A.J. (1984)[11]; Yarbrough, L.W., Tollett, J.L., Montrey, R.D., and Beattie, R.J. (1984)[13]; and Hack, C.A. and Gleiser, C.A. (1982).[14]

Table 97 Mean Control Ranges of Typical Hematology Measurements in New Zealand White Rabbits

Parameters	15–20 Weeks Old	25–40 Weeks Old	1–2 Years Old
Activated partial thromboplastin time (sec)	11.7–14.5	11.3–14.9	10.5–15.8
Erythrocyte count (10^6/mm^3)	5.5–7.0	4.8–6.7	4.9–7.0
Fibrinogen (mg/dl)	125–300	125–300	125–400
Hematocrit (%)	37.0–44.5	37.0–44.5	37.5–44.7
Hemoglobin (g/dl)	12.0–14.7	10.9–14.4	10.5–14.8
Leukocyte count, total (10^3/mm^3)	5.4–11.9	3.6–7.9	4.8–13.5
Mean corpuscular hemoglobin (pg)	20.2–23.0	21.8–24.5	20.4–23.4
Mean corpuscular hemoglobin conc. (g/dl)	32.3–34.9	32.2–34.8	30.0–34.1
Mean corpuscular volume (fl)	61.4–68.6	64.8–69.5	64.8–72.0
Platelet count (10^3/mm^3)	175–500	175–500	200–500
Reticulocyte count (% RBC)	0–2.0	0–2.0	0–3.0
Prothrombin time (sec)	8.2–9.8	8.0–10.0	8.6–10.3

Source: Adapted from Levine, B.S. (1979–1993)[2], Hewitt, C.D., Innes, D.J., Savory, J., and Wills, M.R. (1989)[15]; and Jain (1986).[20]

Table 98 Quantitative Data on Blood Cells in Healthy, Mature, Adult Humans

	Men	Women	Percentage
Hemoglobin (mmol l^{-1})	8.6–10.7	7.4–10.4	
Erythrocytes ($\times 10^{12}$ l^{-1})	4.2–5.5	3.7–5.0	
Hematocrit (l/l)	0.41–0.55	0.36–0.46	
MCV (fl)	85–105	85–105	
MCH (fmol)	1.75–2.23	1.75–2.23	
MCHC (mmol l^{-1})	20–23	20–23	
Thrombocytes ($\times 10^9$ l^{-1})	150–400	150–400	
Leukocytes ($\times 10^9$ l^{-1})			
Total	4.0–11.0	4.0–11.0	100
Lymphocytes	1.5–3.5	1.5–3.6	20–40
Monocytes	0.2–0.8	0.2–0.8	1–6
Neutrophilic granulocytes[a]	2.5–7.5	2.5–7.5	50–75
Eosinophilic granulocytes	0.04–0.44	0.04–0.44	1–3
Basophilic granulocytes	0.01–0.1	0.01–0.1	0–1

Note:

$$MCV = \text{Mean cell volume} = \frac{\text{Hematocrit (l/l)}}{\text{Number of erythrocytes } l^{-1}} \times 10^{15}$$

$$MCH = \text{Mean cell hemoglobin} = \frac{\text{Hemoglobin } \left(\text{mmol } l^{-1}\right)}{\text{Number of erythrocytes } l^{-1}} \times 10^{12}$$

$$MCHC = \text{Mean cell hemoglobin concentration} = \frac{\text{Hemoglobin } \left(\text{mmol } l^{-1}\right)}{\text{Hematocrit (l/l)}}$$

[a] Cells with rod-shaped nuclei: 1–5%; cells with segmented nuclei: 50–70%

From Niesink, R.J.M., deVries, J., and Hollinger, M.A. (1996).[21]

Table 99 24-Hour Mean Urinalysis Data with Standard Deviation (SD) and Standard Error of the Mean (SEM) in Adult Male Rats: Fischer-344, Sprague-Dawley, and Wistar

Parameters	Strain								
	F-344			Sprague-Dawley			Wistar		
	Mean	SD	SEM	Mean	SD	SEM	Mean	SD	SEM
Volume (ml)	5.92	2.15	0.88	14.83	7.63	3.12	12.68	4.06	1.66
Volume (ml/100 g body weight)	1.78	0.556	0.227	2.824	1.339	0.547	2.453	0.761	0.311
Sodium (µEq/ml)	62.7	20.3	8.3	54.3	32.7	13.4	41.67	16.27	6.64
Potassium (µEq/ml)	197.67	32.87	13.42	168.0	75.2	30.7	146.0	37.5	15.3
Chloride (µEq/ml)	105.0	54.5	22.3	64.7	47.5	19.4	60.0	24.9	10.2
Protein (g/dl)	0.4833	0.0983	0.0401	0.5167	0.1941	0.0792	0.3667	0.0816	0.0333
Glucose (mg/dl)	7.33	17.96	7.33	0.00	0.00	0.00	0.00	0.00	0.00
ALP (IU)	154.2	54.4	22.2	87.1	53.7	21.9	141.4	43.4	17.8
LDH (IU)	3.83	9.39	3.83	34.17	83.69	34.17	0.00	0.00	0.00
Osmolality (mOsm/kg)	1312.3	210.5	86.0	1206	497	203	1197	325	133
pH	6.18	0.41	0.17	6.83	0.75	0.31	6.18	0.406	0.17
Creatinine (mg/dl)	144.2	22.8	9.3	142.0	61.9	25.3	165.7	60.7	24.8
Sodium/Cr (µEq/mg Cr)	43.2	124	5.07	35.78	7.88	3.25	25.37	7.55	3.08
Potassium/Cr (µEq/mg Cr)	137.2	11.6	4.72	117.29	15.55	6.38	91.10	16.1	6.59
Chloride/Cr (µEq/mg Cr)	70.3	35.3	14.40	39.5	25.0	10.20	36.9	14.7	5.99
Protein/Cr (g/mg Cr)	0.0039	0.00058	0.00024	0.0038	0.0012	0.00047	0.0023	0.0004	0.00016
Glucose/Cr (mg/mg Cr)	0.05	0.123	0.05	0	0	0	0	0	0

Note: Resting Renal Function — Each animal was placed in an individual metabolism cage for a 24-hour urine sample collection.

Table 100 24-Hour Mean Urinalysis Data with Standard Deviation (SD) and Standard Error of the Mean (SEM) in Adult Female Rats: Fischer-344, Sprague-Dawley, and Wistar

| | Strain | | | | | | | | |
| | F-344 | | | Sprague-Dawley | | | Wistar | | |
Parameters	Mean	SD	SEM	Mean	SD	SEM	Mean	SD	SEM
Volume (ml)	8.82	4.32	1.76	8.43	3.43	1.40	18.22	8.07	3.29
Volume (ml/100 g body weight)	4.93	2.41	.98	2.839	1.119	.457	6.48	2.46	1.00
Sodium (µEq/ml)	152.0	41.4	16.9	155.2	16.2	6.6	81.7	63.5	25.9
Potassium (µEq/ml)	304.0	91.2	36.8	324.2	50.8	20.7	179.7	97.9	40.0
Chloride (µEq/ml)	205.5	61.6	25.2	249.7	78.7	32.1	104.7	79.5	32.5
Protein (g/dl)	0.3333	0.0516	0.0211	0.4667	0.1211	0.0494	0.1833	0.0983	0.0401
Glucose (mg/dl)	9.3	14.5	5.9	8.33	13.05	5.33	0.00	0.00	0.00
ALP (IU)	25.22	11.14	4.55	16.1	11.1	4.5	32.0	24.9	10.2
LDH (IU)	0.00	0.00	0.00	13.83	19.02	7.76	2.50	6.12	2.50
Osmolality (mOsm/kg)	1764	520	212	2286	650	266	1083	428	175
pH	7.00	0.632	0.26	7.83	1.17	0.48	7.50	1.23	.50
Creatinine (mg/dl)	91.8	27.8	11.4	161.5	54.2	22.1	71.50	23.98	9.79
Sodium/Cr (µEq/mg Cr)	169.9	27.7	11.32	105.5	34.6	14.13	120.9	85.0	34.72
Potassium/Cr (µEq/mg Cr)	334.6	27.7	11.32	213.5	47.5	19.39	264.1	129.3	52.77
Chloride/Cr (µEq/mg Cr)	225.6	24.6	10.06	162.8	43.8	17.90	149.9	106.8	43.62
Protein/Cr (g/mg Cr)	0.0040	0.0015	0.00062	0.0031	0.00086	0.00035	0.0027	0.0015	0.0006
Glucose/Cr (mg/mg Cr)	0.0817	0.1266	0.0517	0.0417	0.0646	0.0264	0	0	0

Note: Resting Renal Function — Each animal was placed in an individual metabolism cage for a 24-hour urine sample collection.

Table 101 Comparison of Biochemical Components in Urine of Normal Experimental Animals and Humans

Component (mg/kg body wt/day) or Property	Rat	Rabbit	Cat	Dog	Goat	Sheep
Volume (ml/kg body wt/day)	150–350	20.0–350	10.0–30.0	20.0–167	7.0–40.0	10.0–40.0
Specific gravity	1.040–1.076	1.003–1.036	1.020–1.045	1.015–1.050	1.015–1.062	1.015–1.045
pH	7.30–8.50	7.60–8.80	6.00–7.00	6.00–7.00	7.5–8.80	7.50–8.80
Calcium	3.00–9.00	12.1–19.0	0.20–0.45	1.00–3.00	1.00–3.40	1.00–3.00
Chloride	50.0–75.0	190–300	89.0–130	5.00–15.0	186–376	—
Creatinine	24.0–40.0	20.0–80.0	12.0–30.0	15.0–80.0	10.0–22.0	5.80–14.5
Magnesium	0.20–1.90	0.65–4.20	1.50–3.20	1.70–3.00	0.15–1.80	0.10–1.50
Phosphorous, inorganic	20.0–40.0	10.0–60.0	39.0–62.0	20.0–50.0	0.5–1.6	0.10–0.50
Potassium	50.0–60.0	40.0–55.0	55.0–120	40.0–100	250–360	300–420
Protein, total	1.20–6.20	0.74–1.86	3.10–6.82	1.55–4.96	0.74–2.48	0.74–2.17
Sodium	90.4–110.	50.0–70.0	—	2.00–185	140.–347.	0.80–2.00
Urea nitrogen (g/kg/day)	1.00–1.60	1.20–1.50	0.80–4.00	0.30–0.53	0.14–0.47	0.11–0.17
Uric acid	8.00–12.0	4.00–6.00	0.20–13.0	3.1–6.0	2.00–5.00	2.00–4.00

Table 101 Comparison of Biochemical Components in Urine of Normal Experimental Animals and Humans (Continued)

Component (mg/kg body wt/day) or Property	Swine	Cattle	Horse	Monkey	Man
Volume (ml/kg)	5.00–30.0	17.0–45.0	3.0–18.0	70.0–80.0	8.60–28.6
Specific gravity	1.010–1.050	1.025–1.045	1.020–1.050	1.015–1.065	1.002–1.040
pH	6.25–7.55	7.60–8.40	7.80–8.30	5.50–7.40	4.80–7.80
Calcium	—	0.10–3.60	—	10.0–20.0	0.60–8.30
Chloride	—	10.0–140.	81.0–120	80.0–120.	40.0–180.
Creatinine	20.0–90.0	15.0–30.0	—	20.0–60.0	15.0–30.0
Magnesium	—	2.00–7.00	—	3.20–7.10	0.42–2.40
Phosphorous, inorganic	—	0.01–6.20	0.05–2.00	9.00–20.6	10.0–15.0
Potassium	—	240.–320.	—	160.–245.	16.0–56.0
Protein, total	0.33–1.49	0.25–2.99	0.62–0.99	0.87–2.48	0.81–1.86
Sodium	—	2.00–40.0	—	—	25.0–94.0
Urea nitrogen (g/kg/day)	0.28–0.58	0.05–0.06	0.20–0.80	0.20–0.70	0.20–0.50
Uric acid	1.00–2.00	1.00–4.00	1.00–2.00	1.00–2.00	0.80–3.00

Source: From Mitruka, B.M. and Rawnsley, H.M. (1977).[22] With permission.

References

1. Loeb, W.F. and Quimby, F.W., *The Clinical Chemistry of Laboratory Animals*, Pergamon Press, New York, 1989.
2. Levine, B.S., unpublished data, 1979–1993.
3. Charles River Laboratories, Serum Chemistry Parameters for the Crl:CD®BR Rat, Wilmington, MA, 1993.
4. NIEHS, A Summary of Control Values for F344 Rats and B6C3F1 Mice in 13 Week Subchronic Studies, Program Resources, Inc., Research Triangle Park, NC, 1985.
5. Burns, K.F., Timmons, E.H., and Poiley, S.M., Serum chemistry and hematological values for axenic (germfree) and environmentally associated inbred rats, *Lab. Anim. Sci.*, 21, 415, 1971.
6. Frith, C.H., Suber, R.L., and Umholtz, R., Hematologic and clinical chemistry findings in control BALB/c and C57BL/6 mice, *Lab. Anim. Sci.*, 30, 835, 1980.
7. Wolford, S.T., Schroer, R.A., Gohs, F.X., Gallo, P.P., Brodeck, M., Falk, H.B., and Ruhren, R.J., Reference range data base for serum chemistry and hematology values in laboratory animals, *Toxicol. Environ. Health*, 18, 161, 1986.
8. Clarke, D., Tupari, G., Walker, R., and Smith, G., Stability of serum biochemical variables from Beagle dogs and Cynomolgus monkeys, *Am. Assoc. Clin. Chem.*, Special Issue 17, October 1992.
9. Pickrell, J.A., Schluter, S.J., Belasich, J.J., Stewart, E.V., Meyer, J., Hubbs, C.H., and Jones, R.K., Relationship of age of normal dogs to blood serum constituents and reliability of measured single values, *Am. J. Vet. Res.*, 35, 897, 1974.
10. Kaspar, L.V. and Norris, W.P., Serum chemistry values of normal dogs (Beagles): associations with age, sex and family line, *Lab. Anim. Sci.*, 27, 980, 1977.
11. Kapeghian, L.C. and Verlangieri, A.J., Effects of primaquine on serum biochemical and hematological parameters in anesthetized *Macaca fasicularis*, *J. Med. Primatol.*, 13, 97, 1984.
12. Davy, C.W., Jackson, M.R., and Walker, S., Reference intervals for some clinical chemical parameters in the marmoset (*Callithrix jacchus*): effect of age and sex, *Lab. Anim.*, 18, 135, 1984.

13. Yarbrough, L.W., Tollett, J.L., Montrey, R.D., and Beattie, R.J., Serum biochemical, hematological and body measurement data for common marmosets (*Callithrix jacchus*), *Lab. Anim. Sci.*, 34, 276, 1984.

14. Hack, C.A. and Gleiser, C.A., Hematologic and serum chemical reference values for adult and juvenile Baboons (*Papio* sp.), *Lab. Anim. Sci.*, 32, 502, 1982.

15. Hewett, C.D., Innes, D.J., Savory, J., and Wills, M.R., Normal biochemical and hematological values in New Zealand white rabbits, *Clin. Chem.*, 35, 1777, 1989.

16. Yu, L., Pragay, D.A., Chang, D., and Wicher, K., Biochemical parameters of normal rabbit serum, *Clin. Biochem.*, 12, 83, 1979.

17. Charles River Laboratories, Hematology parameters for the Crl:CD®BR rat, Wilmington, MA, 1993.

18. Bulgin, M.S., Munn, S.L., and Gee, S., Hematologic changes to $4^{1}/_{2}$ years of age in clinically normal Beagle dogs, *J. Am. Vet. Met. Assoc.*, 157, 1004, 1970.

19. Jordan, J.E., Normal laboratory values in Beagle dogs at twelve to eighteen months of age, *Am. J. Vet. Res.*, 38, 409, 1c7.

20. Jain, N.C., *Schalm's Veterinary Hematology*, Lea & Febiger, Philadelphia, 1986.

21. Niesink, R.J.M., deVries, J., and Hollinger, M.A., *Toxicology: Principles and Applications*, CRC Press, Boca Raton, FL, 1996.

22. Mitruka, B.M. and Rawnsley, H.M., *Clinical Biochemical and Hematological Reference Values in Normal Experimental Animals*, Masson Publishing, New York, 1977.

Section 11:
Risk Assessment

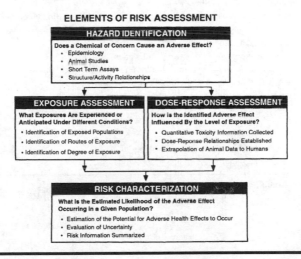

ELEMENTS OF RISK ASSESSMENT

HAZARD IDENTIFICATION

Does a Chemical of Concern Cause an Adverse Effect?
- Epidemiology
- Animal Studies
- Short Term Assays
- Structure/Activity Relationships

EXPOSURE ASSESSMENT

What Exposures Are Experienced or Anticipated Under Different Conditions?
- Identification of Exposed Populations
- Identification of Routes of Exposure
- Identification of Degree of Exposure

DOSE-RESPONSE ASSESSMENT

How is the Identified Adverse Effect Influenced By the Level of Exposure?
- Quantitative Toxicity Information Collected
- Dose-Reponse Relationships Established
- Extrapolation of Animal Data to Humans

RISK CHARACTERIZATION

What Is the Estimated Likelihood of the Adverse Effect Occurring in a Given Population?
- Estimation of the Potential for Adverse Health Effects to Occur
- Evaluation of Uncertainty
- Risk Information Summarized

Figure 6 The four major elements of risk assessment. *Hazard identification* — In this step, a determination is made of whether a chemical of concern is or is not causally linked to a particular health effect. Information can come from human and animal studies, *in vitro* assays, and through analogy to structurally similar chemicals. *Exposure assessment* — involves the characterization of the amount, frequency, and duration of human exposure. Determinations are made of the concentration of hazardous substances in media (i.e., air, water, soil, etc.), magnitude and pathways of exposure, environmental fate, and populations at risk. The purpose of this step is to provide a quantitative estimate of human exposure. *Dose-response assessment* — The relationship between the magnitude of exposure and the occurrence of the expected health effects is determined in this step. Information obtained from animal studies is extrapolated to humans. Generally, different assessments are performed for noncarcinogenic and carcinogenic materials. Along with hazard identification, the major activities of most toxicologists are focused on this portion of the risk assessment process. *Risk characterization* — In this final stage of the risk assessment process, information from the three previous steps is evaluated to produce a determination of the nature and magnitude of human risk. The risk assessment process is completed with a summary of the risk information. The information developed in the risk assessment process will be utilized in the *risk management process* in which decisions are made as to the need for, the degree of, and the steps to be taken to control exposures to the chemical of concern. (U.S. EPA (1989)[1]; National Research Council (1983)[2]; and Hooper, L.D., Oehme, F.W., and Krieger, G.R., Eds. (1992).[3])

Table 102 Typical Factors Considered in a Risk Assessment

- Physical and chemical properties of the chemical
- Patterns of use
- Handling procedures
- Availability and reliability of control measures
- Source and route of exposure under ordinary and extraordinary conditions
- Potential for misuse
- Magnitude, duration, and frequency of exposure
- Nature of exposure (total, dermal, inhalation)
- Physical nature of the exposure (solid, liquid, vapor, etc.)
- Influence of environmental conditions of exposure
- Population exposed
    - Number
    - Sex
    - Health status
    - Personal habits (e.g., smoking)
    - Lifestyles (e.g., hobbies, activities)

Source: From Ballantyne, B. and Sullivan, J.B. (1992).[4]

Table 103   Major Factors that Influence a Risk Assessment

Factor	Effect
Low dose extrapolation	Can involve as many as 50 or more assumptions, each of which introduces uncertainty; often considered the greatest weakness in risk assessment.
Population variation	The use of standard exposure factors can underestimate actual risk to hypersensitive individuals. Addressing the risk assessment to the most sensitive individuals can overestimate risk to the population as a whole.
Exposure variation	The use of modeling and measurement techniques can provide exposure estimates that diverge widely from reality.
Environmental variation	Can affect actual exposures to a greater or lesser degree than assumed to exist.
Multiple exposures	Risk assessments generally deal with one contaminant for which additive, synergistic, and antagonistic effects are unaccounted; can result in underestimate or overestimate of risk.
Species differences	It is generally assumed that humans are equivalent to the most sensitive species; can overestimate or underestimate risk.
Dose based on body weight	Toxicity generally does not vary linearly with body weight but exponentially with body surface area.
Choice of dose levels	Use of unrealistically high dose levels can result in toxicity unlikely to occur at actual exposure levels. The number of animals being studied may be insufficient to detect toxicity at lower doses.
Uncertainty factors	The use of uncertainty factors in attempting to counter the potential uncertainty of a risk assessment can overestimate risk by several orders of magnitude.
Confidence intervals	The upper confidence interval does not represent the true likelihood of an event; can overestimate risk by an order of magnitude or more.
Statistics	Experimental data may be inadequate for statistical analysis. Statistical significance may not indicate biological significance, and a biologically significant effect may not be statistically significant. Statistical significance does not prove causality. Conversely, lack of statistical significance does not prove safety.

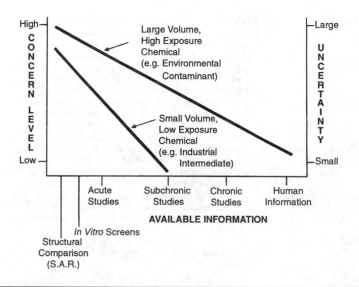

Figure 7 Relationship between the degree of uncertainty associated with the risk assessment of a chemical, the concern for human exposure, and the toxicological information available on the chemical. In practice, the larger the toxicological database available on a chemical of concern ("weight-of-evidence"), the greater the certainty (less uncertainty) that the estimated "safe" exposure level will be protective of individuals exposed to the chemical. Similarly, the concern that the risk assessment will underestimate the risk decreases with a larger toxicological database. Generally, less toxicological information will be required to reduce the concern level and uncertainty associated with a small volume, low-exposure chemical (for which the exposed population is well characterized and the exposures can be controlled) as compared with a large volume, high-exposure chemical.

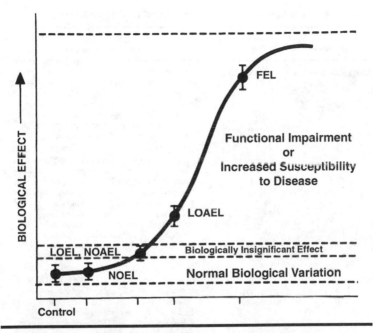

Figure 8   A dose-response curve from a typical toxicology study showing dose-related indices commonly used in risk assessment. A well-designed study should include dose levels that produce a Frank Effect (FEL), a Lowest Observable Adverse Effect (LOAEL), and either a Lowest Observable Effect (LOEL), a No Observable Adverse Effect (NOAEL), or a No Observable Effect (NOEL). A FEL is a dose or exposure level that produces unmistakable *adverse* health effects that cause functional impairment or increased susceptibility to disease; a LOAEL is the lowest dose or exposure level that produces an *adverse* health effect; a LOEL is the lowest dose or exposure level that produces an observable effect, but not to a degree which would be expected to have a significant impact on the health of the animal (the LOEL is sometimes confused with a LOAEL); a NOAEL is the highest dose or exposure level at which no *adverse* health effects are observed which are capable of functional impairment or increase susceptibility to disease (the NOAEL can be equivalent to the LOEL); a NOEL is the highest dose or exposure level at which no effects are observed outside of the range of normal biological variation for the species and strain under study. The effect, if any, observed at the NOEL should not be statistically significant when compared with the control group. (Adapted from Ecobichon, D.J. [1992].[5])

Table 104 Human Data Commonly Used in Risk Assessment

Study Type	Alternative Terms	Comments on Use
Cross-sectional	Prevalence, survey	Random sampling of a population at a given point in time to assess prevalence of a disease. Most useful for studying chronic diseases of high frequency. Cannot measure incidence. Although associations may be drawn with prevalent cases, the temporary and causal order of such associations cannot be determined.
Case-control	Retrospective, dose or case-referent	Compares previous exposure in subjects with disease with one or more groups of subjects without disease. Selection of cases and noncases can be controlled. Exposures cannot be controlled. If exposure data available, an NOEL may be identified. Exposure history may be difficult to reconstruct outside of an occupational setting. Recall and other biases possible due to retrospective evaluation. Allows estimation of relative odds of exposure in cases and controls but not absolute risk.
Cohort	Longitudinal, prospective, incidence	Population or sample of subjects at risk of disease observed through time for outcome of interest. May fail to detect rare outcome. Many factors can be controlled for reduced bias (prospective design). Dose-response curves may be constructed if dose or exposure data is available. Allows estimation of absolute and relative risk.
Clinical trials		Type of cohort study in which investigator controls treatment (exposure). Generally not applicable to environmental issues. Intervention trials in which an exposure is removed or changed (e.g., medication, smoking, diet) are useful for evaluating causality.
Experimental studies		Controlled human exposures generally of low dose and limited exposure time. Used for hazard identification, dose-response, and risk characterization.
Case reports		Suggests nature of acute endpoints. Cannot be used to support absence of hazard.

Source: From Piantadose, S. (1982)[6] and U.S. EPA (1989).[7]

Table 105 Epidemiological Terms

Annual crude death rate $= \dfrac{\text{Total number of deaths during a given year}}{\text{Total polulation at mid-year}} \times 1000$

Annual specific death rate $= \dfrac{\text{Total number of deaths in a specific group during a given year}}{\text{Total population in the specific group at mid-year}}$

$\times 1000$

Proportional mortality rate $= \dfrac{\text{Total number of deaths in a specific group}}{\text{Total number of deaths}} \times 100$

Infant mortality rate (IMR) $= \dfrac{\text{Infant deaths}}{\text{Total live births}}$

Standard mortality rate (SMR) $= \dfrac{\text{Observed deaths}}{\text{Expected deaths}}$

Cause-of-death ratio $= \dfrac{\text{Deaths from a specific cause over a period of time}}{\text{Total deaths due to all causes in the same time period}} \times 100$

Incidence rate $= \dfrac{\text{Number of new cases over a period of time}}{\text{Population at risk}}$

Prevalence rate $= \dfrac{\text{Number of existing cases at a point in time}}{\text{Total population}}$

Relative risk (risk ratio) $= \dfrac{\text{Incidence among the exposed}}{\text{Incidence among the nonexposed}}$

Attributal risk (risk difference) $=$ Incidence among the exposed − incidence among the nonexposed

Relative odds ratio $= \dfrac{\text{Number of exposed individuals with disease}}{\text{Number of exposed individuals without disease}}$

$\times \dfrac{\text{Number of nonexposed individuals without disease}}{\text{Number of nonexposed individuals with disease}}$

Source: From Selevan, S.G. (1993)[8]; Hallenbeck, W.H. and Cunningham, K.M. (1986)[9]; and Gamble and Battigelli (1978).[10]

Table 106   The Duration of Studies in Experimental Animals and Time Equivalents in the Human

Species	Duration of Study in Months				
	1	**3**	**6**	**12**	**24**
Percent of Lifespan					
Rat	4.1	12	25	49	99
Rabbit	1.5	4.5	9	18	36
Dog	0.82	2.5	4.9	9.8	20
Pig	0.82	2.5	4.9	9.8	20
Monkey	0.55	1.6	3.3	6.6	13
Human Equivalents (in months)					
Rat	34	101	202	404	808
Rabbit	12	36	72	145	289
Dog	6.5	20	40	81	162
Pig	6.5	20	40	81	162
Monkey	4.5	13	27	61	107

Source: Adapted from Paget, G.E., Ed. (1970).[11] From Ecobichon, D.J. (1992).[12] With permission.

Table 107 Comparative Mammalian Reference Values for Relative Dose Calculations

Species	Average Lifespan (yr)	Body Weight (kg)	Food Consumption (g/day)	Food Consumption Factor[a]	Water Consumption (ml/day)	Inhalation Rate (m³/day)
Human	70	70	2000	0.028	2000	20
Mouse	1.5–2	0.03	4	0.13	6	0.052
Rat	2	0.35	18	0.05	50	0.29
Hamster	2.4	0.14	12	0.083	27	0.13
Guinea pig	4.5	0.84	34	0.040	200	0.40
Rabbit	7.8	3.8	186	0.049	410	?
Cat	17	3	90	0.030	220	1.2
Dog	12	12.7	318	0.025	610	4.3
Monkey (Rhesus)	18	8	320	0.040	530	5.4

[a] Fraction of body weight consumed per day as food.

Source: Adapted from U.S. EPA (1985).[13]

Table 108 Reference Comparative Physiological Values

Parameter	Mouse	Rat	Human
Tissue Perfusion (% of cardiac output)			
Brain	7.5 (2.0–13.0)	1.2	14.0 (13.0–15.0)
Heart	4.4 (2.8–6.0)	2.9	3.3 (2.6–4.0)
Kidney	24.8 (14.6–35.0)	17.8	22.0
Liver (total)	21.0	18.6 (17.0–26.0)	26.5 (26.0–27.0)
Liver (arterial only)	8.4	6.7	—a
Viscera	30.3	26.3	30.0
Adipose tissue	—a	4.5 (4.0–5.0)	4.7 (4.5–5.0)
Tissue Volume (% of body weight)			
Heart	0.4	0.5	0.6
Kidney	1.5	0.9 (0.9–1.0)	1.1 (0.4–1.5)
Liver	5.0 (4.0–5.9)	4.0 (3.7–4.2)	3.0 (2.4–4.0)
GI tract	6.8	4.3 (3.0–5.5)	3.8 (3.0–4.5)
Fat	7.6 (4.0–9.8)	8.4 (7.0–9.0)	15.5 (9.0–23.1)
Blood	7.6	7.2 (4.9–9.0)	7.2
Muscle	59.0 (45.0–73.0)	59.0 (50.0–73.0)	52.4 (43.4–73.0)
Skin	14.5	16.0	4.3
Marrow	2.7	—a	2.5 (2.1–2.8)
Skeletal tissue	9.0	—a	—a
Cardiac Output			
Absolute (liters/min)	0.0129 (0.110–0.160)	0.1066 (0.0730–0.1340)	5.59 (4.60–6.49)
Relative (liters/min·kg)	0.535 (0.440–0.711)	0.327 (0.248–0.646)	0.080 —a
Alveolar Ventilation (liters/min)			
	0.026 (0.012–0.039)	0.080 (0.075–0.085)	4.6 (4.0–5.8)
Minute Volume			
Absolute (liters/min)	0.038 (0.024–0.052)	0.169 (0.057–0.336)	7.4 (6.0–9.0)
Relative (liters/min·kg)	1.533 (1.239–1.925)	0.780 (0.142–2.054)	0.089 (0.014–0.127)

Table 108   Reference Comparative Physiological Values (Continued)

Parameter	Mouse	Rat	Human
	Respiratory Frequency (breaths/min)		
	171	117	14
	(100–213)	(60–153)	(10–16)

Note: Mean of reported values. Brackets contain range of reported values from which mean was calculated. Absence of range indicates value was from a single report. Values presented are for unanesthetized animals.

a No data found.

Source: Data derived from U.S. EPA (1988).[14]

Table 109   Body Fluid Volumes for Men and Women

Parameter	Adult Males[a]		Adult Female[b]	
	Volume (liters)	% of Bodyweight	Volume (liters)	% of Bodyweight
Total body water	45.0	60	33.0	55
Extracellular water	11.25	15	9.0	15
Intracellular water	33.75	45	24.0	40
Total blood volume	5.4	7.2	4.3	7.2
Plasma volume	3.0	—	2.6	—
Erythrocyte volume	2.4	—	1.7	—

a Volumes calculated for an adult male with a body weight of 75 kg and a hematocrit of 45%.

b Volumes calculated for an adult female with a body weight of 60 kg and a hematocrit of 40%.

Source: Adapted from Plowchalk, D., Meadows, M.J., and Mattinson, D.R. (1993).[15]

Table 110 Comparative Mammalian Organ Weights (g/100 g body weight)

Species	Brain	Heart	Adrenals	Kidneys	Lungs	Liver	Spleen	Testes
Human	1.96	0.42	0.02	0.41	0.73	2.30	0.25	0.04
Mouse	1.35	0.68	0.02	2.60	0.66	5.29	0.32	0.62
Rat	0.46	0.32	0.01	0.70	0.40	3.10	0.20	0.92
Monkey (Rhesus)	2.78	0.38	0.02	—	1.89	2.09	—	—
Dog	0.59	0.85	0.01	0.30	0.94	2.94	0.45	0.15
Rabbit	0.40	0.35	0.02	0.70	0.53	3.19	0.04	0.13
Hamster	0.88	0.47	0.02	0.53	0.46	5.16	—	—
Guinea pig	1.33	0.53	0.07	1.17	1.18	5.14	0.21	0.65
Cat	0.77	0.45	0.02	1.07	1.04	2.59	0.29	0.07

Table 111 EPA Recommended Human Exposure Values for Use in Risk Assessments

Body weight[a]	
Young child (2–5 yr)	13.2 kg
Older child (6 yr)	20.8 kg
Adult	70 kg
Lifespan	75 yr
Exposed skin surface area[b]	
Typical adult	0.20 m²
Reasonable worst case	0.53 m²
Swimming or bathing (50th percentile)	1.94 m² (male) 1.69 m² (female)
Inhalation rate[c]	
8-hr work shift	10 m³ day
Average adult	20 m³ day
Reasonable worst case	30 m³ day
Drinking water ingestion rate	
Adult (average)	1.4 liters/day
Adult (reasonable worst case)	2.0 liters/day
Infant (≤10 kg)	1.0 liters/day

Table 111   EPA Recommended Human Exposure Values for Use in Risk Assessments (Continued)

Food Consumption Rates		
Adult total food consumption		2000 g/day
a.	Beef consumption (homegrown)	
	Typical	44 g/day
	Reasonable worst case	75 g/day
	Average total (homegrown and other)	100 g/day
b.	Dairy consumption (homegrown)	
	Typical	160 g/day
	Reasonable worst case	300 g/day
	Average total (homegrown and other)	400 g/day
c.	Fish consumption (sport fish)	
	Average (50th percentile)	30 g/day
	90th percentile	140 g/day
d.	Fruit consumption (homegrown)	
	Typical	28 g/day
	Reasonable worst case	42 g/day
	Average total (homegrown and other)	140 g/day
e.	Vegetable consumption (homegrown)	
	Typical	50 g/day
	Reasonable worst case	80 g/day
	Average total (homegrown and other)	200 g/day
Soil ingestion rates		
Children less than 7 yr (average)		0.2 g/day
Children less than 7 yr (90th percentile)		0.8 g/day
Showering		
Median		7 min
90th percentile		12 min
(A 5-min shower is estimated to use 40 gallons of water)		

[a] See Table 38 in Derelanko, M.J. and Hollinger, M.A., *CRC Handbook of Toxicology*, CRC Press, Boca Raton, FL, 1995, for more detailed information.

[b] See Tables 40 and 42 in Derelanko, M.J. and Hollinger, M.A., *CRC Handbook of Toxicology*, CRC Press, Boca Raton, FL, 1995, for more detailed information.

[c] See Table 44 in Derelanko, M.J. and Hollinger, M.A., *CRC Handbook of Toxicology*, CRC Press, Boca Raton, FL, 1995, for more detailed information.

Source: From U.S. EPA (1989).[16]

Table 112 Constants for Estimating Surface Area (A) of Mammals

Species	Constant (K)
Rat	9.6
Mouse	9.0
Rabbit	10.0
Guinea pig	9.0
Monkey	11.8
Dog	11.0
Cat	8.7

$A = KW^{2/3}$ where A = surface area (cm²); K = constant; W = body weight (g).

Source: Data derived from Spector, W.S., Ed. (1956).[17]

Table 113 Median Total Body Surface Area (m²) for Humans by Age

Age (years)	Males	Females
3–5	0.728	0.711
6–8	0.931	0.919
9–11	1.16	1.16
12–14	1.49	1.48
15–17	1.75	1.60
Adult	1.94	1.69

Source: Adapted from U.S. EPA (1989).[16]

Table 114 Relationship Between Body Weight and Body Surface Area in a Number of Vertebrates

Species	Weight (g)	Surface Area (cm²)
Mouse	20	46
Rat	200	325
Guinea pig	400	565
Rabbit	1,500	1,270
Cat	2,000	1,380
Monkey	4,000	2,980
Dog	12,000	5,770
Man	70,000	18,000

From Niesink, R.J.M., deVries, J., and Hollinger, M.A. (1996).[18]

Table 115 Summary of Human Inhalation Rates for Men, Women, and Children by Activity Level (m³/hour)

	Resting[a]	Light[b]	Moderate[c]	Heavy[d]
Adult male	0.7	0.8	2.5	4.8
Adult female	0.3	0.5	1.6	2.9
Average adult[e]	0.5	0.6	2.1	3.9
Child, age 6	0.4	0.8	2.0	2.4
Child, age 10	0.4	1.0	3.2	4.2

Note: Values of inhalation rates for males, females, and children presented in this table represent the mean of values reported for each activity level in USEPA (1985).[13]

[a] Includes watching television, reading, and sleeping.

[b] Includes most domestic work, attending to personal needs and care, hobbies, and conducting minor indoor repairs and home improvement.

[c] Includes heavy indoor cleanup, performance of major indoor repairs and alterations, and climbing stairs.

[d] Includes vigorous physical exercise and climbing stairs carrying a load.

[e] Derived by taking the mean of the adult male and adult female values for each activity level.

Source: From U.S. EPA (1989).[16]

Table 116 Risk Assessment Calculations

1. Human Equivalent Dose (HED)

$$HED = \left(Animal\ dose\right) \times \left(\frac{Human\ body\ weight}{Animal\ body\ weight}\right)^{1/3}$$

2. ppm ↔ mg/m³ Conversion

$$ppm = \frac{\left(mg/m^3\right) \times \left(R\right)}{\left(MW\right)}$$

where ppm = exposure concentration as ppm; mg/m³ = exposure concentration as mg/m³, R = universal gas constant (24.5 at 25°C and 760 mmHg); MW = molecular weight.

3. Airborne Concentration to Equivalent Oral Dose

$$EOD = \frac{\left(C\right) \times \left(EL\right) \times \left(MV\right) \times \left(AF\right) \times \left(10^{-6}\right)}{\left(BW\right)}$$

where EOD = equivalent oral dose (mg/kg); C = concentration of substance in air (mg/m³); EL = exposure length (min); MV = minute volume, species specific (ml/min); AF = absorption factor (fraction of inhaled substance absorbed), default = 1; 10^{-6} = m³ ↔ ml conversion; BW = body weight (kg).

4. Oral Dose to Equivalent Airborne Concentration

$$EAC = \frac{\left(OD\right) \times \left(BW\right)}{\left(MV\right) \times \left(AF\right) \times \left(EL\right) \times \left(10^{-6}\right)}$$

where EAC = equivalent airborne concentration (mg/m³); OD = oral dose (mg/kg); BW = body weight (kg); MV = minute volume, species specific (ml/min); AF = absorption factor, fraction of inhaled substance absorbed; (default = 1) EL = exposure length (min); 10^{-6} = m³ ↔ ml conversion.

5. Lifetime Exposure (hr)

Lifetime = (hours exposed) × (days exposed) × (weeks exposed) × (years exposed)
exposure   per day   per week   per week   per year

Note: Methods 3 and 4 are crude approximations in that the time period will be set and protracted for the inhalation and may be either bolus for gavage studies or averaged over the entire day (feeding and drinking water) for oral. They also assume that there will be no chemical reactivity associated with oral administration, no portal entry effects and that the target organ effects will be the same regardless of the route of administration.

Table 116   Risk Assessment Calculations (Continued)

6. Exposure from Ingestion of Contaminated Water

$$LADD = \frac{(C) \times (CR) \times (ED) \times (AF)}{(BW) \times (TL)}$$

where LADD = lifetime average daily dose (mg/kg/day); C = concentration of contaminant in water (mg/liter); CR = water consumption rate (liters/day); ED = exposure duration (days); AF = absorption factor (fraction of ingested contaminant absorbed) default = 1 (dimensionless); BW = body weight (kg); TL = typical lifetime (days).

7. Exposure from Dermal Contact with Contaminated Water

$$LADD = \frac{(C) \times (SA) \times (EL) \times (AR) \times (ED) \times (SV) \times (10^{-9})}{(BW) \times (TL)}$$

where LADD = lifetime average daily dose (mg/kg/day); C = concentration of contaminant in water (mg/liter); SA = surface area of exposed skin (cm²); EL = exposure length (min/day); AR = absorption rate (μg/cm²/min); SV = specific volume of water (1 liter/kg); ED = exposure duration (days); 10^{-9} = kg ↔ μg conversion); BW = body weight (kg); TL = typical lifetime (days).

8. Exposure from Ingestion of Contaminated Soil

$$LADD = \frac{(C) \times (CR) \times (ED) \times (AF) \times (FC) \times (10^{-6})}{(BW) \times (TL)}$$

where LADD = lifetime average daily dose (mg/kg/day); C = concentration of contaminant in soil (mg/kg); CR = soil consumption rate (mg/day); ED = exposure duration (days); AF = absorption factor (fraction of ingested contaminant absorbed) default = 1 (dimensionless); FC = fraction of total soil from contaminated source; 10^{-6} = kg ↔ mg conversion; BW = body weight (kg); TL = typical lifetime (days).

9. Exposure from Dermal Contact with Contaminated Soil

$$LADD = \frac{(C) \times (SA) \times (BF) \times (FC) \times (SDF) \times (ED) \times (10^{-6})}{(BW) \times (TL)}$$

Table 116   Risk Assessment Calculations (Continued)

where LADD = lifetime average daily dose (mg/kg/day); C = concentration of contaminant in soil (mg/kg); SA = surface area of exposed skin (cm²); BF = bioavailability factor (percent absorbed/day); FC = fraction of total soil from contaminated source; SDF = soil deposition factor; amount deposited per unit area of skin (mg/cm²/day); ED = exposure duration (days); BW = body weight (kg); TL = typical lifetime (days).

10. **Exposure from Inhalation of Contaminated Particles in Air**

$$LADD = \frac{(C) \times (PC) \times (IR) \times (RF) \times (EL) \times (AF) \times (ED) \times (10^{-6})}{(BW) \times (TL)}$$

where LADD = lifetime average daily dose (mg/kg/day); C = concentration of contaminant on particulate (mg/kg); PC = particulate concentration in air (mg/m³); IR = inhalation rate (m³/hr); RF = respirable fraction of particulates; EL = exposure length (hr/day); AF = absorption factor (fraction of inhaled contaminant absorbed) default = 1; ED = exposure duration (days); 10^{-6} = kg ↔ mg conversion; BW = body weight (kg); TL = typical lifetime (days).

11. **Exposure from Inhalation of Vapors**

$$LADD = \frac{(C) \times (IR) \times (EL) \times (AF) \times (ED)}{(BW) \times (TL)}$$

where LADD = lifetime average daily dose (mg/kg/day); C = concentration of contaminant in air (mg/m³); IR = inhalation rate (m³/hr); EL = exposure length (hr/day); AF = absorption factor (fraction of inhaled contaminant absorbed) default = 1; ED = exposure duration (days); BW = body weight (kg); TL = typical lifetime (days).

12. **Calculation of an RfD**

$$RfD = \frac{(NOAEL)}{(UFs) \times (MF)}$$

where RfD = reference dose (mg/kg/day); UFs = uncertainty factors — generally multiples of 10 (although 3 and 1 are occasionally used, depending on the strength and quality of the data). The following uncertainty factors are usually used:

UF 10 Accounts for variation in the general population. Intended to protect sensitive subpopulations (e.g., elderly, children).

10 Used when extrapolating from animals to humans. Intended to account for interspecies variability between humans and animals.

Table 116   Risk Assessment Calculations (Continued)

10 Used when an NOAEL is derived from a subchronic rather than a chronic study in calculating a chronic RfD.

10 Applied when an LOAEL is used instead of an NOAEL. Intended to account for the uncertainty in extrapolating from LOAELs to NOAELs.

MF = modifying factor; multiple of 1 to 10; intended to reflect a professional qualitative assessment of the uncertainty in the critical study from which the NOAEL is derived as well as the overall quality of the database. Accounts for the uncertainty not addressed by the UFs.

13.   Estimating an LD_{50} of a Mixture

$$\frac{1}{\text{Predicted LD}_{50}} = \frac{Pa}{\text{LD}_{50} \text{ of Component a}} + \frac{Pb}{\text{LD}_{50} \text{ of Component b}}$$
$$+ \cdots \frac{Pn}{\text{LD}_{50} \text{ of Component n}}$$

where P = fraction of components in the mixture.

14.   Time-Weighted Average (TWA) for an 8-hr Workday

$$\text{TWA} = \frac{C_1 T_1 + C_2 T_2 + \ldots C_n T_n}{8}$$

where C_n = concentration measured during a period of time (<8 hr); T_n = duration of the period of exposure in hours at concentration C_n ($\Sigma T = 8$).

15.   Risk for Noncarcinogens (Hazard Index)

$$\text{Risk} = \frac{\text{MDD}}{\text{ADI}}$$

If: Risk > 1, a potential risk exists which may be significant.
     Risk < 1, risk is insignificant.

where MDD = maximum daily dose; and ADI = acceptable daily intake.

16.   Lifetime Risk for Carcinogens
Risk = (LADD) × (SF)

If risks = 10^{-6}, risk is insignificant; 10^{-6}–10^{-4}, possible risk; 10^{-4}, risk may be significant.

Table 116   Risk Assessment Calculations (Continued)

where LADD = lifetime average daily dose (mg/kg/day); SF = slope factor or cancer potency factor $(mg/kg/day)^{-1}$ (chemical and route specific).

17. Total Risk from a Single Contaminant via Multiple Exposure Pathways

Total = Σ Risks from all exposure pathways

Example:

Total risk (from a contaminant in water) = (Risk from ingestion) + (Risk from showering) + (Risk from swimming).

18. Total Risk from Multiple Contaminants via a Single Exposure Pathway

Total risk = Σ Risks from all contaminants in the media

Example:

Total risk from contaminants, A, B, and C in water = Total risk from contaminant A + Total risk from contaminant B + Total risk from contaminant C

Note: For evaluation 17 and 18, total risk < 1 is insignificant; total risk > 1 may be significant. Both of these methods are extremely conservative and can greatly overestimate risk.

Source: From U.S. EPA (1989)[16]; Paustenbach, D.J. and Leung, H.-W. (1993)[19]; Environ Corporation (1990)[20]; U.S. EPA (1989)[21]; and Lynch, J.R. (1979).[22]

References

1. U.S. Environmental Protection Agency, General Quantitative Risk Assessment Guidance for Non-Cancer Health Effects, ECAP-CIN-538M, 1989; as cited in Hooper et al.[3]

2. National Research Council, *Risk Assessment in the Federal Government*, National Academy Press, Washington, D.C., 1983.

3. Hooper, L.D., Oehme, F.W., and Krieger, G.R., Risk assessment for toxic hazards, in *Hazardous Materials Toxicology: Clinical Principles of Environmental Health*, Sullivan, J.B. and Krieger, G.R., Eds., Williams & Wilkins, Baltimore, MD, 1992, chap. 7.

4. Ballantyne, B. and Sullivan, J.B., Basic principles of toxicology, in Hazardous *Materials Toxicology: Clinical Principles of Environmental Health*, Sullivan, J.B. and Krieger, G.R., Eds., Williams & Wilkins, Baltimore, MD, 1992, chap. 2.

5. Ecobichon, D.J., *The Basis of Toxicity Testing*, CRC Press, Boca Raton, FL, 1992, chap. 7.

6. Piantadose, S., Epidemiology and principles of surveillance regarding toxic hazards in the environment, in *Hazardous Materials Toxicology: Clinical Principles of Environmental Health*, Sullivan, J.B. and Krieger, G.R., Eds., Williams & Wilkins, Baltimore, MD, 1992, chap. 6.

7. U.S. Environmental Protection Agency, *Interim Methods for the Development of Inhalation Reference Doses*, Blackburn, K., Dourson, M., Erdreich, L., Jarabek, A.M., and Overton, J., Jr., Eds., Environmental Criteria and Assessment Offices, EPA/600/8-88/066F, 1989.

8. Selevan, S.G., Epidemiology, in *Occupational and Environmental Reproductive Hazards: A Guide for Clinicians*, Paul, M., Ed., Williams & Wilkins, Baltimore, 1993, chap. 9.

9. Hallenbeck, W.H. and Cunningham K.M., Qualitative evaluation of human and animal studies, in Quantitative *Risk Assessment for Environmental and Occupational Health*, Lewis Publishers, Chelsea, MI, 1986, chap.3.

10. Gamble, J.F. and Battigelli, M.C., Epidemiology, in *Patty's Industrial Hygiene and Toxicology*, 3rd rev., ed. vol. I, Clayton, G.D. and Clayton, F.E., Eds., John Wiley & Sons, New York, 1978, chap. 5.

11. Paget, G.E., Ed., *Methods in Toxicology*, Blackwell Scientific Publishers, Oxford, 1970, 49.

12. Ecobichon, D.J., *The Basis of Toxicity Testing*, CRC Press, Boca Raton, FL, 1992, chap. 4.

13. U.S. Environmental Protection Agency, Development of Statistical Distributions or Ranges of Standard Factors Used in Exposure Assessments, Office of Health and Environmental Assessments, EPA No. 600/8-85-010, NTIS, PB85-242667, 1985.

14. U.S. Environmental Protection Agency, *Reference Physiological Parameters in Pharmacokinetic Modeling*, Arms, A.D. and Travis, C.C., Eds., Office of Risk Analysis, EPA No., 600/6-88/004, 1988.

15. Plowchalk, D., Meadows, M.J., and Mattinson, D.R., Comparative approach to toxicokinetics, in *Occupational and Environmental Reproductive Hazards, A Guide for Clinicians*, Paul, M., Ed., Williams and Wilkins, Baltimore, 1993, chap. 3.

16. U.S. Environmental Protection Agency, *Exposure Factors Handbook*, Konz, J.J., Lisi, K., Friebele, E., and Dixon, D.A., Eds., Office of Health and Environmental Assessments, EPA No. 600/8-89/043, 1989.

17. Spector, W.S., Ed., *Handbook of Biological Data*, W.B. Saunders, Philadelphia, 1956, 175.

18. Niesink, R.J.M., deVries, J., and Hollinger, M.A., *Toxicology: Principles and Applications*, CRC Press, Boca Raton, FL, 1996.

19. Paustenbach, D.J. and Leung, H.-W., Techniques for assessing the health risk of dermal contact with chemicals in the environment, in *Health Risk Assessment: Dermal and Inhalation Exposure and Absorption of Toxicants*, Wang, R.G.M., Knaak, J.B., and Maibach, H.I., Eds., CRC Press, Boca Raton, FL, 1993, chap. 23.

20. Environ Corporation, *Risk Assessment Guidance Manual*, AlliedSignal, Inc., Morristown, NJ, 1990.

21. U.S. Environmental Protection Agency, *Risk Assessment Guidance for Superfund, Vol. 1: Health Evaluation Manual*, Office of Emergency and Remedial Response, EPA No. 540/1-89/002, 1989.

22. Lynch, J.R., Measurement of worker exposure, in *Patty's Industrial Hygiene and Toxicology, Vol. III: Theory and Rationale of Industrial Hygiene Practice*, Cralley, L.V. and Cralley, L.J., Eds., John Wiley & Sons, New York, 1979, chap. 6.

Section 12:
Regulatory Toxicology

Table 117   Combined Tabulation of Toxicity Classes

		Various Routes of Administration			
Toxicity Rating	Commonly Used Term	LD_{50} Single Oral Dose Rats	Inhalation 4-hr Vapor Exposure Mortality 2/6–4/6 Rats	LD_{50} Skin Rabbits	Probable Lethal Dose for Man
1	Extremely toxic	≤1 mg/kg	<10 ppm	≤5 mg/kg	A taste, 1 grain
2	Highly toxic	1–50 mg	10–100 ppm	5–43 mg/kg	1 teaspoon, 4 cc
3	Moderately toxic	50–500 mg	100–1000 ppm	44–340 mg/kg	1 ounce, 30 gm
4	Slightly toxic	0.5–5 g	1000–10,000 ppm	0.35–2.81 g/kg	1 cup, 250 gm
5	Practically nontoxic	5–15 g	10,000– 100,000 ppm	2.82–22.59 g/kg	1 quart, 1000 gm
6	Relatively harmless	>15 g	>100,000 ppm	>22.6 g/kg	>1 quart

Source: Adapted from Hodge, H.C. and Sterner, J.H. (1949).[1] With permission.

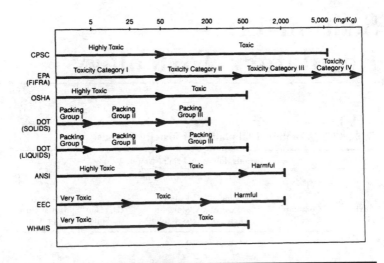

Figure 9 Toxicity classifications based on rat acute oral LD$_{50}$. CPSC = Consumer Product Safety Commission; EPA = U.S. Environmental Protection Agency; (FIFRA = Federal Insecticide, Fungicide and Rodenticide Act); OSHA = U.S. Occupational Safety and Health Administration; DOT = U.S. Department of Transportation; ANSI = American National Standards Institute; EEC = European Economic Community; WHMIS = Workplace Hazardous Materials Information System (Canada). Use the following example of the DOT (solids) classification as an aid for interpreting the values of this figure: Packing Group I (≤5 mg/kg); Packing Group II (>5 mg/kg to ≤50 mg/kg); Packing Group III (>50 mg/kg to ≤200 mg/kg). (Adapted from Schurger, M.G. and McConnell, F., Eastman Chemicals, Kingsport, TN, 1989.[2] With permission.)

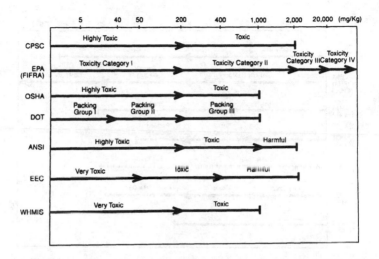

Figure 10   Toxicity classifications based on rabbit or rat acute dermal LD$_{50}$. CPSC = Consumer Product Safety Commission; EPA = U.S. Environmental Protection Agency; (FIFRA = Federal Insecticide, Fungicide and Rodenticide Act); OSHA = U.S. Occupational Safety and Health Administration; DOT = U.S. Department of Transportation; ANSI = American National Standards Institute; EEC = European Economic Community; WHMIS = Workplace Hazardous Materials Information System (Canada). Refer to the legend for Figure 9 for an aid to interpreting the values of this figure. (Adapted from Schurger, M.G. and McConnell, F., Eastman Chemicals, Kingsport, TN, 1989.[2] With permission.)

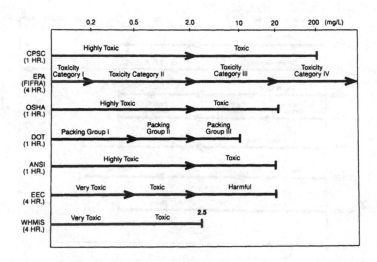

Figure 11   Toxicity classifications based on rat acute inhalation LC$_{50}$. CPSC = Consumer Product Safety Commission; EPA = U.S. Environmental Protection Agency; (FIFRA = Federal Insecticide, Fungicide and Rodenticide Act); OSHA = U.S. Occupational Safety and Health Administration; DOT = U.S. Department of Transportation; ANSI = American National Standards Institute; EEC = European Economic Community; WHMIS = Workplace Hazardous Materials Information System (Canada). Refer to the legend for Figure 9 for an aid to interpreting the values of this figure. (Adapted from Schurger, M.G. and McConnell, F., Eastman Chemicals, Kingsport, TN, 1989.[2] With permission.)

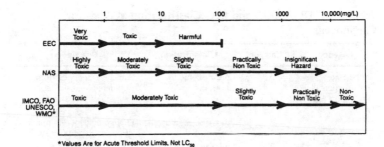

*Values Are for Acute Threshold Limits, Not LC₅₀

Figure 12 Toxicity classifications based on acute fish LC_{50}. EEC = European Economic Community; NAS = U.S. National Academy of Sciences; IMCO = Inter-Government Maritime Consultive Organization; FAO = Food and Agriculture Organization; UNESCO = United Nations Educational, Scientific and Cultural Organization; WMO = World Meteorological Organization. Refer to the legend for Figure 9 for an aid to interpreting the values of this figure.

Table 118   EPA, IARC, and EEC Classification Systems for Carcinogens

Agency	Category	Classification	Description
United States Environmental Protection Agency (EP)	A	Carcinogenic to humans	Sufficient evidence from epidemiology studies to support a casual association
	B1	Probably carcinogenic to humans	Limited evidence in humans from epidemiology studies
	B2	Probably carcinogenic to humans	Sufficient evidence from animal studies but inadequate or no data in humans
	C	Possibly carcinogenic to humans	Limited or equivocal evidence from animal studies but inadequate or no data in humans
	D	Not classifiable as to human carcinogenicity	Inadequate or no data from animals and inadequate or no data in humans
	E	Evidence of noncarcinogenicity for humans	No evidence of carcinogenicity in at least two animal species and no evidence in humans
International Agency for Research on Cancer (IARC)	1	Carcinogenic to humans	Sufficient epidemiological evidence for carcinogenicity in humans
	2A	Probably carcinogenic to humans	Sufficient evidence from animal studies and limited evidence in humans
	2B	Possibly carcinogenic to humans	Sufficient evidence from animal studies but inadequate evidence in humans
			— or —
			Limited evidence in humans but insufficient evidence in animals
	3	Not classifiable as to human carcinogenicity	Inadequate data to classify
	4	Not carcinogenic	Sufficient evidence of noncarcinogenicity in humans and/or animals

Table 118   EPA, IARC, and EEC Classification Systems for Carcinogens (Continued)

Agency	Category	Classification	Description
European Economic Community (EEC)	1	Known to be carcinogenic to humans	Sufficient evidence to establish a casual association between human exposure and cancer
	2	Regarded as if carcinogenic to humans	Sufficient evidence to provide a strong presumption that human exposure may result in cancer. Based on long-term animal studies and/or other relevant information
	3	Causes concern due to possible carcinogenic effects	Inadequate information to make a satisfactory assessment. Some evidence from animal studies but insufficient to place in category 2.

Source: Adapted from Ecobichon, D.J. (1992)[3] and European Economic Community (EC) (1993).[4]

Table 119   Major U.S. Regulatory Agencies Having Involvement with Toxicology

Agency	Agency Description	Coverage	Authority to Require Toxicity Testing/Reporting		
			Premarket Testing	Testing by Manufacturer	Reporting of Data
Food and Drug Administration (FDA)	A unit of the department of Health and Human Services	• Drugs and foods	X	X	X
		• Food additives and cosmetics	X	X	—
Environmental Protection Agency (EPA)	Independent agency, not a part of a cabinet department	• Pesticides	X	X	X
		• Industrial chemicals	(X)[a]	X	X
		• Air pollutants	—	—	—
		• Industrial waste	—	X	X
Occupational Safety and Health Administration (OSHA)	Unit of the Department of Labor	• Occupational Exposure	—	—	X
Consumer Product Safety Commission (CPSC)	Independent commission	• Consumer products	—	—	X

[a]   Can require testing based on available data.

Table 120 EPA Categories of Concern with Brief Description of Toxicological Concerns

Category	Concern
Acid chlorides	Toxic to aquatic organisms. Concern is greater if the log octanol/water partition coefficient (log K_{ow}) > 8 or if molecular weight (mol. wt.) < 1000.
Dyes: acid	Many of these dyes are toxic to fish and aquatic organisms, particularly if the substance is water soluble and mol. wt. is around 1000 or less.
Dyes: cationic	Water-soluble cationic dyes are toxic to fish, daphnids, and algae, whereas poorly soluble dyes tend to be toxic only to algae.
Acrylamides	The acrylamides of greatest concern are those with a labile substituent, (e.g., methylol acrylamides) that may release acrylamide *per se* under metabolic conditions. Members of this class are considered potential carcinogens, heritable mutagens, developmental and reproductive toxicants, and are potential neurotoxins. Structures with an acrylamide equivalent wt. ≥ 5000 are presumed *not* to pose a hazard under *any* condition.
Acrylates and methacrylates	There is concern for carcinogenicity and neurotoxicity. Ecotoxicity is also a concern, particularly if the log of the oct/water partition coefficient (log P) < 5. Concerns typically confined to species with mol. wt. < 1000.
Aliphatic amines	Can be highly toxic to all groups of freshwater organisms. Generally, members of this concern category will have mol. wt. < 1000.
Alkoxy silanes	The "typical" substance of concern is a polymer with a substantial fraction of species with mol. wt. < 1000 and pendant trimethoxy or triethoxysilane groups. There is a concern for irreversible lung toxicity if such substances are inhaled. They are also toxic to algae and aquatic invertebrates.
Dyes: aminobenzothiazole AZO	There are oncogenicity and mutagenicity concerns. There is also potential for liver, thyroid, and neurotoxicity. Ecotoxicity concerns generally relate to chronic toxicity.
Carboxylic acid anhydrides	Potential for pulmonary sensitization; also developmental or reproductive toxicity (if mol. wt. < 500)
Anilines	Acute toxicity is expected if log K_{ow} < 7.38 and mol. wt. < 1000.

Table 120   EPA Categories of Concern with Brief Description of Toxicological Concerns (Continued)

Category	Concern
Dianilines (Must have *at least* two phenyl rings with a bridging carbon, oxygen, nitrogen, or sulfur. Each terminal phenyl ring must have a primary amino group [or a group that can be readily metabolized to a primary amino group])	Potential carcinogens and mutagens; also potential retinotoxic agents; and also potential reproductive and systemic toxicants.
Benzotriazoles	Only compounds with mol. wt. < 1000 are expected to manifest toxicity. Acute toxicity is expected if log K_{ow} ≤ 5.0 and mol. wt. < 1000. Only chronic toxicity is expected when log K_{ow} > 5.0 and < 8.0, and mol. wt. < 1000.
Borates	All boron hydrides are highly toxic for mammals. The major environmental hazard concerns for this category are for chronic toxicity toward fish and toxicity toward green algae.
Surfactants: cationic	Cationic surfactants are biocidal to a wide array of species in the environment. Little ecotoxicity is expected when the carbon chain length exceeds 22 carbons.
Surfactants: nonionic	Acute aquatic toxicity increases with the hydrophobic chain length up to 16–18 carbons. Aquatic toxicity is decreased with increasing number of ethoxylate or propoxylate groups.
Surfactants: anionic	Toxic to a wide variety of aquatic organisms.
Diazoniums (aromatic only)	Those with mol. wt. < 1000 are of particular concern. The concern is acute and chronic ecotoxicity.
Dithiocarbamates (and their metal salts)	The concern is ecotoxicity. Generally, members of this category will have mol. wt. < 1000.
Epoxides	Health concerns for epoxides are for cancer and reproductive effects. Structures with epoxy equivalent weights ≥ 1000 are presumed *not* to pose a hazard under *any* conditions.
Esters	Compounds with molecular weights > 1000 are not of concern. The concern is aquatic toxicity.

Table 120   EPA Categories of Concern with Brief Description of Toxicological Concerns (Continued)

Category	Concern
Ethylene glycol ethers	Short-chain ethylene glycol ethers are absorbed by all routes of exposures and have caused irritation of skin, eyes, and mucous membranes; hemolysis, bone-marrow damage, and leukopenia of both lymphocytes and granulocytes; direct and indirect kidney damage; liver damage; immunotoxicity; and central nervous system depression. They are also developmental and reproductive toxicants.
Hydrazines and related compounds	There are concerns for carcinogenicity and chronic effects to liver, kidney, and blood. There are also ecotoxicity concerns.
Hindered amines	May be toxic to the immune system, liver, blood, male reproductive system, and gastrointestinal tract.
Imides	Compounds with mol. wt. < 1000 are of greater concern. The primary toxicity concern is for aquatic organisms.
Isocyanates (includes any substances containing *two or more* isocyanate groups)	Concern because of potential dermal and pulmonary sensitization and other lung effects. Aromatic isocyanates may be potential carcinogens. Structures with an isocyanate equivalent weight of > 5000 are presumed *not* to pose a hazard under *any* conditions.
β-Naphthylamines (monosulfonated)	Potential carcinogens and mutagens. Concern is restricted to those compounds where the sulfonate or sulfatoethylsulfone group is on the ring *distal* to the β-amino group.
Neutral organics	"Neutral organics" are believed to be environmentally toxic. The molecular weights of neutral organics of concern are generally < 1000 and the octanol/water partition coefficients (log P) are < 8.
Nickel compounds	Nickel produces acute and chronic toxicity to aquatic organisms overt a wide range of concentrations.
Peroxides	Members of this category may be carcinogenic.
Phenols	Compounds of greater concern have mol. wt. < 1000. The primary concern is for acute and chronic toxicity to aquatic organisms.
Polyanionic polymers (and monomers)	Compounds must be water soluble or water self-dispersing to be in this category. The concern is toxicity to aquatic organisms (ecotoxicity).
Polycationic polymers	The concern is ecotoxicity. The polymers must be water soluble or water dispersible and the molecular weights are generally > 300.

Table 120   EPA Categories of Concern with Brief Description of Toxicological Concerns (Continued)

Category	Concern
Polynitroaromatics	Concern is for compounds with mol. wt. < 1000. The concern is for aquatic or ecotoxicity.
Stilbene, derivatives of 4,4-bis(triazin-2-ylamino)-	There are developmental reproductive toxicity concerns.
Substituted triazines	The concern is for ecotoxicity.
Vinyl esters	An example of this category is vinyl acetate. Major concerns are oncogenicity, neurotoxicity, reproductive toxicity, and environmental toxicity.
Vinyl sulfones	There is concern for carcinogenicity based on the potent mutagenicity of methylvinyl sulfone.
Soluble complexes of zinc	Zinc can produce acute and chronic toxicity to freshwater organisms over a range of concentrations.
Zirconium compounds	Soluble salts of Zr are known to be moderately toxic to algae and fish. Only water-soluble Zr compounds with mol. wt. < 1000 are expected to be toxic.

Source: From U.S. EPA (1992).[5]

Table 121   Criteria Defining "High-Exposure" Chemicals

- Production greater than 100,000 kg
- More than 1000 workers exposed
- More than 100 workers exposed by inhalation to greater than 10 mg/kg/day
- More than 100 workers exposed by inhalation to 1–10 mg/day for more than 100 days/year
- More than 250 workers exposed by routine dermal contact for more than 100 days/year
- Presence of the chemical in any consumer product in which the physical state of the chemical in the product and the manner of use would make exposure likely
- More than 70 mg/year of exposure via surface water
- More than 70 mg/year of exposure via air
- More than 70 mg/year of exposure via groundwater
- More than 10,000 kg/year release to environmental media
- More than 1000 kg/year total release to surface water after calculated estimates of treatment

Source: From U.S. EPA (1988).[6]

Table 122 Substances Generally Recognized as Safe

Section 21 CFR Part 182 lists the following items as Generally Recognized as Safe (GRAS)[a]

Multiple-Purpose GRAS Food Substances

Citric acid
Glutamic acid
Glutamic acid hydrochloride
Hydrochloric acid
Phosphoric acid
Sodium acid pyrophosphate
Aluminum sulfate
Aluminum ammonium sulfate
Aluminum potassium sulfate
Aluminum sodium sulfate
Caffeine
Calcium citrate
Calcium phosphate
Caramel

Glycerin
Methylcellulose
Monoammonium glutamate
Monopotassium glutamate
Potassium citrate
Silica aerogel
Sodium carboxymethylcellulose
Sodium caseinate
Sodium citrate
Sodium phosphate
Sodium aluminum phosphate

Sodium tripolyphosphate
High fructose corn syrup
Triethyl citrate

Dietary Supplements

Ascorbic acid
Linoleic acid
Biotin
Calcium carbonate
Calcium citrate
Calcium glycerophosphate
Calcium oxide
Calcium pantothenate
Calcium phosphate
Calcium pyrophosphate
Carotene
Choline bitartrate
Choline chloride
Copper gluconate
Ferric phosphate
Ferric pyrophosphate
Ferric sodium pyrophosphate
Ferrous gluconate
Ferrous lactate
Ferrous sulfate
Inositol
Iron reduced

Dietary Supplements (Cont'd)

Magnesium oxide
Magnesium phosphate
Magnesium sulfate
Magnesium chloride
Manganese citrate
Manganese gluconate
Manganese glycerophosphate

Sequestrants

Citric acid
Sodium acid phosphate
Calcium citrate
Calcium diacetate
Calcium hexametaphosphate
Monobasic calcium phosphate
Dipotassium phosphate
Disodium phosphate
Isopropyl citrate
Monoisopropyl citrate
Potassium citrate
Sodium citrate
Sodium gluconate
Sodium hexametaphosphate
Sodium metaphosphate
Sodium phosphate
Sodium pyrophosphate

Table 122   Substances Generally Recognized as Safe (Continued)

Sequestrants (Cont'd)

Tetra sodium
  pyrophosphate
Sodium
  tripolyphosphate
Stearyl citrate

Stabilizers

Chondrus extract

Anticaking Agents

Aluminum calcium
  silicate
Calcium silicate
Magnesium silicate
Sodium aluminosilicate
Sodium calcium
  aluminosilicate
  hydrated
Tricalcium silicate

Chemical Preservatives

Ascorbic acid
Erythorbic acid
Sorbic acid

Thiodipropionic
  acid
Ascorbyl palmitate
Butylated
  hydroxyanisole
Butylated
  hydroxytoluene
Calcium ascorbate
Calcium sorbate
Dilauryl
  thiodipropionate

**Chemical Preservatives
(Cont'd)**

Potassium
  bisulfite
Potassium
  metabisulfite
Potassium sorbate
Sodium ascorbate
Sodium bisulfite
Sodium metabisulfite
Sodium sorbate
Sodium sulfite
Sulfur
  dioxide
Tocopherols

Dietary Supplements

Manganese sulfate
Manganous oxide
Niacin
Niacinamide
D-Pantothenyl alcohol
Potassium chloride
Potassium
  glycerophosphate
Pyridoxine
  hydrochloride
Riboflavin
Riboflavin-5-
  phosphate
Sodium
  pantothenate
Sodium phosphate
Thiamine hydrochloride
Thiamine
  mononitrate

Tocopherols

α-Tocopherol
  acetate
Vitamin A
Vitamin A acetate
Vitamin A palmitate
Vitamin B_{12}
Vitamin D_2
Vitamin D_3
Zinc
  chloride
Zinc gluconate
Zinc oxide
Zinc stearate
Zinc sulfate

Nutrients

Ascorbic acid
Biotin
Calcium citrate
Calcium phosphate
Calcium
  pyrophosphate
Choline
  bitartrate
Choline chloride
Manganese
  hypophosphite
Sodium
  phosphate
Tocopherols
α-Tocopherol acetate
Zinc
  chloride

[a]   21 CFR Part 182, chap. 1 (4-1-92 Edition) 181, 33.

Table 123   European Notification of a New Substance: Information and Test Data Required

Annual Total	Cumulative Total	Data Requirements (Refer to Table 124)
<10 kg		Exempt
10–100 kg		Annex VII C
100–1000 kg	500 kg	Annex VII B
>1,000 kg (1 tonne)	5000 kg	Annex VII A
>10 tonnes	50 tonnes	Level 1 (may be required[a])
>100 tonnes	500 tonnes	Level 1
>1000 tonnes	5000 tonnes	Level 2

[a] Testing at 10/50 tonnage thresholds will depend on the nature of the chemical, its uses, and the results of existing tests.

Source: From Brooker, P.C. (1993).[7] With permission.

Table 124 Data Requirements for European Notification

Annex VII C
Supply at 10–100 kg/yr

Flash point/flammability
Acute toxicity (oral or inhalation)

Annex VII B
(Supply at 100–1000 kg/yr or 500 kg cumulative)

Melting point/boiling point	Eye irritation
Water solubility	Skin sensitization
Partition coefficient (*n*-octanol/water)	Ames
Flashpoint/flammability	
Vapor pressure (may be required	Biodegradation
	Daphnia acute toxicity test (may be required
Acute toxicity (oral or inhalation)	
Skin irritation	

Annex VII A
"The Base Set"
(Supply at >1000 kg/yr or 5000 kg cumulative

Melting point/boiling point	Flash point flammability
Relative density	Explosive properties
Vapor pressure	Self-ignition temperature
Surface tension	Oxidizing properties
Water solubility	Granulometry
Partition coefficient (*n*-octanol/water)	
	Ames test
Acute toxicity (2 routes)	*In vitro* cytogenetics
Skin irritation	Reproductive toxicity screen
Eye irritation	Toxicokinetic assessment (derived from base set data)
Skin sensitization	
28-Day repeat dose toxicity	
	Biodegradation
Acute toxicity for fish	Hydrolysis as a function of pH
Acute toxicity for *Daphnia*	Soil adsorption/desorption screen
Algal growth inhibition	
Bacterial inhibition	

Table 124 Data Requirements for European Notification (Continued)

Level 1 Studies[a] Annex VIII

(Supply at >10[b] or 100 tonnes/yr or 50[b] tonnes cumulative)

Analytical method development	21-Day *Daphnia* toxicity
Physicochemical properties of thermal decomposition products	Further fish toxicity studies
	Bioaccumulation study
	Test on higher plants
Fertility study (one generation)	Earthworm toxicity
Teratology study	Inherent biodegradation
Subchronic/chronic toxicity study	Further adsorption/desorption
Additional mutagenicity studies	
Basic toxicokinetics	

Level 2 Studies[c] Annex VIII

(Supply at >1000 tonnes/yr or 5000 tonnes cumulative)

Chronic toxicity study	Additional test for accumulation, degradation, and mobility
Carcinogenicity study	
Fertility study (2-generation)	Additional test for adsorption/desorption
Developmental toxicity (peri and postnatal)	Further fish toxicity studies
Teratology study (different species from level 1)	Bird toxicity studies
	Toxicity studies with other organisms
Biotransformation	
Pharmacokinetics	
Additional test to investigate organ or system toxicity	

[a] Studies required at level 1 are on a negotiated basis. Negotiations begin once a trigger tonnage has been exceeded. Studies chosen will be based on 1) the quantity supplied, 2) the results of the Base-Set Tests and 3) the degree of exposure to humans and the environment.

[b] Testing at the 10/50 tonnage thresholds will depend on the nature of the chemical, its uses, and the results of earlier tests.

[c] Studies required at level 2 are on a negotiated basis. Negotiations begin once a trigger tonnage has been exceeded. Studies chosen will be based on: 1) the quantity supplied, 2) the results of earlier tests, and 3) the degree of exposure to humans and the environment.

Source: From Brooker, P.C. (1993).[7] With permission.

Table 125   Risk (R) Phrases Used in the European Community

R1	Explosive when dry
R2	Risk of explosion by shock, friction, fire, or other sources of ignition
R3	Extreme risk of explosion by shock, friction, fire, or other sources of ignition
R4	Forms very sensitive explosive metallic compounds
R5	Heating may cause an explosion
R6	Explosive with or without contact with air
R7	May cause fire
R8	Contact with combustible material may cause fire
R9	Explosive when mixed with combustible material
R10	Flammable
R11	Highly flammable
R12	Extremely flammable
R14	Reacts violently with water
R15	Contact with water liberates extremely flammable gases
R16	Explosive when mixed with oxidizing substances
R17	Spontaneously flammable in air
R18	In use may form flammable/explosive vapor-air mixture
R19	May form explosive peroxides
R20	Harmful by inhalation
R21	Harmful in contact with skin
R22	Harmful if swallowed
R23	Toxic by inhalation
R24	Toxic in contact with skin
R25	Toxic if swallowed
R26	Very toxic by inhalation
R27	Very toxic in contact with skin
R28	Very toxic if swallowed
R29	Contact with water liberates toxic gas
R30	Can become highly flammable in use
R31	Contact with acids liberates toxic gas
R32	Contact with acids liberates very toxic gas
R33	Danger of cumulative effects
R34	Causes burns
R35	Causes severe burns
R36	Irritating to the eyes
R37	Irritating to the respiratory system
R38	Irritating to the skin
R39	Danger of very serious irreversible effects

Table 125   Risk (R) Phrases Used in the European Community (Continued)

R40	Possible risk of irreversible effects
R41	Risk of serious damage to the eyes
R42	May cause sensitization by inhalation
R43	May cause sensitization by skin contact
R44	Risk of explosion if heated under confinement
R45	May cause cancer
R46	May cause heritable genetic damage
R48	Danger of serious damage to health by prolonged exposure
R49	May cause cancer by inhalation
R50	Very toxic to aquatic organisms
R51	Toxic to aquatic organisms
R52	Harmful to aquatic organisms
R53	May cause long-term adverse effects in the aquatic environment
R54	Toxic to flora
R55	Toxic to fauna
R56	Toxic to soil organisms
R57	Toxic to bees
R58	May cause long-term adverse effects to the environment
R59	Dangerous for the ozone layer
R60	May impair fertility
R61	May cause harm to the unborn child
R62	Possible risk of impaired fertility
R63	Possible risk of harm to the unborn child
R64	May cause harm to breast-fed babies
Combination of particular risks	
R14/15	Reacts violently with water, liberating extremely flammable gases
R15/29	Contact with water liberates toxic, extremely flammable gas
R20/21	Harmful by inhalation and in contact with skin
R20/21/22	Harmful by inhalation, in contact with skin, and if swallowed
R20/22	Harmful by inhalation and if swallowed
R21/22	Harmful in contact with skin and if swallowed
R23/24	Toxic by inhalation and in contact with skin
R23/24/25	Toxic by inhalation, in contact with skin, and if swallowed
R23/25	Toxic by inhalation and if swallowed
R24/25	Toxic in contact with skin and if swallowed
R26/27	Very toxic by inhalation and in contact with skin
R26/27/28	Very toxic by inhalation, in contact with skin and if swallowed

Table 125   Risk (R) Phrases Used in the European Community (Continued)

R26/28	Very toxic by inhalation and if swallowed
R27/28	Very toxic in contact with skin and if swallowed
R36/37	Irritating to eyes, respiratory system
R36/37/38	Irritating to eyes, respiratory system, and skin
R36/38	Irritating to eyes and skin
R37/38	Irritating to respiratory system and skin
R39/23	Toxic: danger of very serious irreversible effects through inhalation
R39/23/24	Toxic: danger of very serious irreversible effects through inhalation and in contact with skin
R39/23/24/25	Toxic: danger of very serious irreversible effects through inhalation, in contact with skin, and if swallowed
R39/23/25	Toxic: danger of very serious irreversible effects through inhalation and if swallowed
R39/24	Toxic: danger of very serious irreversible effects in contact with skin
R39/24/25	Toxic: danger of very serious irreversible effects in contact with skin and if swallowed
R39/25	Very Toxic: danger of very serious irreversible effects if swallowed
R39/26	Very Toxic: danger of very serious irreversible effects through inhalation
R39/26/27	Very Toxic: danger of very serious irreversible effects through inhalation and in contact with skin
R39/26/27/28	Very Toxic: danger of very serious irreversible effects through inhalation, in contact with skin, and if swallowed
R39/26/28	Very Toxic: danger of very serious irreversible effects through inhalation and if swallowed
R39/27	Very Toxic: danger of very serious irreversible effects in contact with skin
R39/27/28	Very Toxic: danger of very serious irreversible effects in contact with skin and if swallowed
R39/28	Very Toxic: danger of very serious irreversible effects if swallowed
R40/20	Harmful: possible risk of irreversible effects through inhalation
R40/20/21	Harmful: possible risk of irreversible effects through inhalation and in contact with skin
R40/20/21/22	Harmful: possible risk of irreversible effects through inhalation, in contact with skin, and if swallowed
R40/20/22	Harmful: possible risk of irreversible effects through inhalation and if swallowed
R40/22	Harmful: possible risk of irreversible effects if swallowed
R40/21	Harmful: possible risk of irreversible effects in contact with skin
R40/21/22	Harmful: possible risk of irreversible effects in contact with skin and if swallowed
R42/43	May cause sensitization by inhalation and skin contact

Table 125   Risk (R) Phrases Used in the European Community (Continued)

R48/20	Harmful: danger of serious damage to health by prolonged exposure through inhalation
R48/20/21	Harmful: danger of serious damage to health by prolonged exposure through inhalation and in contact with skin
R48/20/21/22	Harmful: danger of serious damage to health by prolonged exposure through inhalation, in contact with skin, and if swallowed
R48/20/22	Harmful: danger of serious damage to health by prolonged exposure through inhalation and if swallowed
R48/21	Harmful: danger of serious damage to health by prolonged exposure in contact with skin
R48/21/22	Harmful: danger of serious damage to health by prolonged exposure in contact with skin and if swallowed
R48/22	Harmful: danger of serious damage to health by prolonged exposure if swallowed
R48/23	Toxic: danger of serious damage to health by prolonged exposure through inhalation
R48/23/24	Toxic: danger of serious damage to health by prolonged exposure through inhalation and in contact with skin
R48/23/24/25	Toxic: danger of serious damage to health by prolonged exposure through inhalation, in contact with skin, and if swallowed
R48/23/25	Toxic: danger of serious damage to health by prolonged exposure through inhalation and if swallowed
R48/24	Toxic: danger of serious damage to health by prolonged exposure in contact with skin
R48/24/25	Toxic: danger of serious damage to health by prolonged exposure in contact with skin and if swallowed
R48/25	Toxic: danger of serious damage to health by prolonged exposure if swallowed
R50/53	Very toxic to aquatic organisms, may cause long-term adverse effects in the aquatic environment
R51/53	Toxic to aquatic organisms; may cause long-term adverse effects in the aquatic environment
R52/53	Harmful to aquatic organisms; may cause long-term adverse effects in the aquatic environment

References

1. Hodge, H.C. and Sterner, J.H., *Am. Ind. Hyg. Assoc. Q.*, 10, 4, 1949.
2. Schurger, M.G. and McConnell, F., Eastman Chemicals, Kingsport, TN, 1989.
3. Ecobichon, D.J., *The Basis of Toxicity Testing*, CRC Press, Boca Raton, FL, 1992, chap. 2.
4. European Economic Community (EEC), 18th Adaptation to Technical Progress, Directive 93/21/EEC, *Off. J. Eur. Econ. Commun.*, 36, No. L110A/61, May 5, 1993.
5. U.S. Environmental Protection Agency, New Chemicals Program (NCP) Categories of Concern, September 1992.
6. U.S. Environmental Protection Agency, Reported in *Pesticide and Toxic Chemical News*, Oct. 19, p. 34, 1988.
7. Brooker, P.C., Huntingdon Research Centre, Ltd., Huntingdon, U.K., personal communication, 1993.

Section 13: General Information

Table 126   Comparison of Physiological Parameters for Different Body Organs

Organ	Weight (kg)	Percent of Body Volume	Percent Water	Blood Flow (ml/min)	Plasma Flow (ml/min)	Blood Flow (ml/kg)	Blood Flow Fraction
Adrenal glands		0.03	—	25	15		
Blood	5.4	7	83	5000			
Bone	10	16	22	250	150		
Brain	1.5	2	75	700	420	780	
Fat	10	10	10	200	120		0.05
Heart	0.3	0.5	79	200	120	250	
Kidneys	0.3	0.4	83	1100	660	1200	
Liver	1.5	2.3	68	1350	810	1500	0.25
Portal				1050	630		
Arterial				300	180		
Lungs	1.0	0.7	79	5000	3000		
Muscle	30	42	76	750	450	900	0.19
Skin	5	18	72	300	180	250	
Thyroid gland	0.03	0.03	—	50	30		
Total body		100	60	5000	3000		

Note: data are for hypothetical 70-kg human.

Source: Adapted from Illing (1989).[1]

Table 127 Comparison of the Blood Flow/Perfusion and Oxygen Consumption of Liver, Lung, Intestine, and Kidney of the Rat *In Vivo* and in Organ Perfusion

Parameter (unit)	Liver	Lung	Intestine	Kidney
In vivo				
Blood flow (ml min^{-1})	13–20	55–70	5–8	4–6
Blood pressure S/D (torr)[a]	150/100	25/10	150/100	150/100
pO$_2$-arterial (torr)	95	40	95	95
pO$_2$-venous (torr)	40	100	50	70
O$_2$-consumption (µl min^{-1})	500–800	From air	40–160	100–200
In perfusion				
Perfusion flow (ml min^{-1})	30–50	50	6	20–35
Perfusion pressure (torr)	100–120	10–20	100–120	100–120
pO$_2$-arterial (torr)	600	600	400	600
pO$_2$-venous (torr)	200	?	180	400
Max. O$_2$-supply[b] (µl min^{-1})	380–630	?	120[c]	120–220

Note: These values are indications of the most common values measured for the various organs in a rat of 250 to 300 g. The figures provided for the kidney apply to a single kidney. The values measured in organ perfusions may differ greatly, depending on the setup, method of gassing, etc.

[a] S = systolic; D = diastolic.

[b] Calculated from pO$_2$-arterial, pO$_2$-venous, and perfusion flow.

[c] With 20% FC-43 emulsion in KRB; other figures apply to KRB buffer without erythrocytes or oxygen carrier (KRB = Krebs-Ringer buffer).

From Niesink, R.J.M., deVries, J., Hollinger, M.A. (1996).[2]

Table 128 Comparison of Physiological Characteristics of Experimental Animals and Humans

Species	Body Wt (kg)	Surface Area (cm²)	Energy Metabolism[a]		Cardiac Function					Arterial Blood Pressure (mm Hg)	
			cal/kg/day	cal/m²/day	Heart Wt. (g/100g)	Heart Rate (beats/min)	Stroke Vol. (ml/beat)	Cardiac Output (ℓ/min)	Cardiac Index (l/m²/m)	Systolic	Diastolic
Rat	0.1–0.5	0.03–0.06	120–140 (B)	760–905 (B)	0.24–0.58	250–400	1.3–2.0	0.015–0.079	1.6	88–184	58–145
Rabbit	1–4	0.23	47	810	0.19–0.36	123–330	1.3–3.8	0.25–0.75	1.7	95–130	60–90
Monkey	2–4	0.31	49 (B)	675	0.34–0.39	165–240	8.8	1.06	—	137–188	112–152
Dog	5–31	0.39–0.78	34–39 (B)	770–800 (B)	0.65–0.96	72–130	14–22	0.65–1.57	2.9	95–136	43–66
Man	54–94	1.65–1.83	23–26 (B)	790–910 (B)	0.45–0.65	41–108	62.8	5.6	3.3	92–150	53–90
Pig	100–250	2.9–3.2	14–17 (B)	1100–1360 (B)	0.25–0.40	55–86	39–43	5.4	4.8	144–185	98–120
Ox	500–800	4.2–8.0	15 (B)	1635 (B)	0.31–0.53	40–58	244	146	—	121–166	80–120
Horse	650–800	5.8–8.0	25 (R)	2710–2770 (R)	0.39–0.94	23–70	852	188	4.4	86–104	43–86

[a] B = basal; R = resting.

Source: From Mitruka, B.M. and Rawnsley, H.M. (1977).[3] With permission.

Table 129   Comparison of Certain Physiological Values of Experimental Animals and Humans

Species	Body Temperature (°C)	Whole Blood Volume (ml/kg body wt.)	Plasma Volume (mg/kg body wt.)	Plasma pH	Plasma CO_2 Content (mM/l)	CO_2 Pressure (mmHg)
Mouse	36.5 ± 0.70	74.5 ± 17.0	48.8 ± 17.0	7.40 ± 0.06	22.5 ± 4.50	40.0 ± 5.40
Rat	37.3 ± 1.40	58.0 ± 14.0	31.3 ± 12.0	7.35 ± 0.09	24.0 ± 4.70	42.0 ± 5.70
Hamster	36.0 ± 0.50	72.0 ± 15.0	45.5 ± 7.50	7.39 ± 0.08	37.3 ± 2.50	59.0 ± 5.00
Guinea pig	37.9 ± 0.95	74.0 ± 7.00	38.8 ± 4.50	7.35 ± 0.09	22.0 ± 6.60	40.0 ± 9.80
Rabbit	38.8 ± 0.65	69.4 ± 12.0	43.5 ± 9.10	7.32 ± 0.03	22.8 ± 8.60	40.0 ± 11.5
Chicken	41.4 ± 0.25	95.5 ± 24.0	65.6 ± 12.5	7.52 ± 0.04	23.0 ± 2.50	26.0 ± 4.50
Cat	38.6 ± 0.70	84.6 ± 14.5	47.7 ± 12.0	7.43 ± 0.03	20.4 ± 3.50	36.0 ± 4.60
Dog	38.9 ± 0.65	92.6 ± 29.5	53.8 ± 20.1	7.42 ± 0.04	21.4 ± 3.90	38.0 ± 5.50
Monkey	38.8 ± 0.80	75.0 ± 14.0	44.7 ± 13.0	7.46 ± 0.06	29.3 ± 3.8	44.0 ± 4.8
Pig	39.3 ± 0.30	69.4 ± 11.5	41.9 ± 8.90	7.40 ± 0.08	30.2 ± 2.5	43.0 ± 5.60
Goat	39.5 ± 0.60	71.0 ± 14.0	55.5 ± 13.0	7.41 ± 0.09	25.2 ± 2.8	50.0 ± 9.40
Sheep	38.8 ± 0.80	58.0 ± 8.50	41.9 ± 12.0	7.48 ± 0.06	26.2 ± 5.00	38.0 ± 8.50
Cattle	38.6 ± 0.30	57.4 ± 5.00	38.8 ± 2.50	7.38 ± 0.05	31.0 ± 3.0	48.0 ± 4.80
Horse	37.8 ± 0.25	72.0 ± 15.0	51.5 ± 12.0	7.42 ± 0.03	28.0 ± 4.00	47.0 ± 8.50
Man	36.9 ± 0.35	77.8 ± 15.0	47.9 ± 8.70	7.39 ± 0.06	27.0 ± 2.00	42.0 ± 5.00

Source: From Mitruka, B.M. and Rawnsley, H.M. (1977).[3] With permission.

Table 130   Tissue Localization of Xenobiotic-Metabolizing Enzymes

Relative Amount	Tissue
High	Liver
Medium	Lung, kidney, intestine
Low	Skin, testes, placenta, adrenals
Very low	Nervous system tissues

Table 131   Metabolic Phase I and Phase II Reactions

Phase I	Phase II
Oxidation	Glucuronidation
Reduction	Glucosidation
Hydrolysis	Ethereal sulfation
Isomerization	Methylation
Others	Acetylation
	Amino acid conjugation
	Glutathione conjugation
	Fatty acid conjugation
	Condensation

Table 132   Cytochrome P450 Gene Families

Gene Symbol	Trivial Name	Inducer	Characteristic Reaction
CYP1A	IA	Polycyclic aromatic hydrocarbons	Benzo[a]pyrene hydroxylation
CYP2A	IIA		Steroid hydroxylation
CYP2B	IIB	Phenobarbital	Benzphetamine demethylation
CYP2C	IIC		Steroid hydroxylation
CYP2D	IID		Debrisoquine hydroxylation
CYP2E	IIE	Ethanol	Ethanol oxidation
CYP3A	IIIA	Steroids and phenobarbital	Steroid hydroxylation
CYP4A	IVA	Hypolipidemic agents	Lauric acid hydroxylation
CYP4B	IVB		
CYP11A	XIA		Cholesterol side chain cleavage
CYP11B	XIB		Deoxycortisol 11β-hydroxylation
CYP17	XVII		Pregnenolone 17α-hydroxylation
CYP19	XIX		Androgen conversion to estrogens
CYP21	XXI		Progesterone 21-hydroxylation

Source: Adapted from Sipes, I.G. and Gandolfi, A.J. (1992).[4]

Table 133 First-Order Process of a Xenobiotic

					Time after Uptake (hours)				
	0	1	2	3	4	5	6	7	8
Chemical eliminated (mg)	0	20	16	12.8	10	8.2	6.6	5.2	4.2
Chemical remaining (mg)	100	80	64	51	41	33.0	26	21	16.8
Chemical eliminated		20/100	16/80	12.8/63.8	10/51	8.1/41.2	6.6/32.6	5.2/26.2	4.3/21.0
(% of remaining)		20	20	20	20	20	20	20	20

Table 134 Xenobiotic Steady State and Half-Life

Number of Half-Life	Xenobiotic Steady State (%)	Xenobiotic Left in Body (%)
1	50.00	50.00
2	75.00	25.00
3	87.50	12.50
4	93.75	6.25
5	96.87	3.13

Note: It takes 4 to 5 half-life values to reach the steady state.

Table 135   Greek Alphabet

Greek Letter		Greek Name	English Equivalent	Greek Letter			Greek Name	English Equivalent
A	α	Alpha	a	N	ν		Nu	n
B	β	Beta	b	Ξ	ξ		Xi	x
Γ	γ	Gamma	g	O	o		Omicron	o
Δ	δ	Delta	d	Π	π		Pi	p
E	ε	Epsilon	ĕ	P	ρ		Rho	r
Z	ζ	Zeta	z	Σ	σ	$\bar{e}$	Sigma	s
H	η	Eta	$\bar{e}$	T	τ		Tau	t
Θ	θ	ϑ	Theta	th	Y	υ		Upsilon	u
I	ι	Iota	i	Φ	φ	φ	Phi	ph
K	κ	Kappa	k	X	χ		Chi	ch
Λ	λ	Lambda	l	Ψ	ψ		Psi	ps
M	μ	Mu	m	Ω	ω		Omega	$\bar{o}$

Source: From Beyer, W.H. (1991).[5]

Table 136   Prefixes and Symbols for Decimal Multiples and Submultiples

Factor	Prefix	Symbol
10^{18}	exa	E
10^{15}	peta	P
10^{12}	tera	T
10^{9}	giga	G
10^{6}	mega	M
10^{3}	kilo	k
10^{2*}	hecto	h
10^{1*}	deka	da
10^{-1*}	deci	d
10^{-2*}	centi	c
10^{-3}	milli	m
10^{-6}	micro	μ
10^{-9}	nano	n
10^{-12}	pico	p
10^{-15}	femto	f
10^{-18}	atto	a

Note: The preferred multiples and submultiples listed above change the quantity by increments of 10^{3} or 10^{-3}. The exceptions to these recommended factors are indicated by the asterisk.

Source: From Beyer, W.H. (1991).[5]

Table 137 Conversion of Human Hematological Values from Traditional Units into SI Units

Constituent	Traditional Units	Multiplication Factor	SI Units
Clotting time	Minutes	0.06	ks
Prothrombin time	Seconds	1.0	arb. unit
Hematocrit (erythrocytes, volume fraction)	%	0.01	1
Hemoglobin	g/100 ml	0.6205	mmol/l
Leukocyte count (leukocytes, number concentration)	per mm^3	10^6	10^9/l
Erythrocyte count (erythrocytes, number concentration)	million per mm^3	10^6	10^{12}/l
Mean corpuscular volume (MCV)	μ^3	1.0	fl
Mean corpuscular hemoglobin (MCH) (Erc-Hemoglobin, amount of substance)	pg	0.06205	fmol
Mean corpuscular hemoglobin concentration (MCHC) (Erc-Hemoglobin, substance concentration)	%	0.6205	mmol/l
Erythrocyte sedimentation rate	mm/hour	1.0	arb. unit
Platelet count (blood platelets, number concentration)	mm^3	10^6	10^9/l
Reticulocyte count (Erc-Reticulocytes, number fraction)	% red cells	0.01	1

Note: To convert xenobiotic concentrations to or from SI units: Conversion factor (CF) = 1000/mol. wt.; conversion *to* SI units: μg/ml × CF = μmol/l; conversion *from* SI units: μmol/l ÷ CF = μg/ml

Source: From Young, D.S. (1975).[6]

Table 138 Conversion of Laboratory Values from Traditional Units into SI Units

Constituent	Traditional Units	Multiplication Factor	SI Units
Amylase	units/l	1.0	arb. unit
Bilirubin (direct)	mg/100 ml	43.06	μmol/l
Conjugated	mg/100 ml	17.10	μmol/l
Total	mg/100 ml	17.10	μmol/l
Calcium	mg/100 ml	0.2495	mmol/l
Carbon dioxide	mEq/l	1.0	mmol/l
Chloride	mEq/l	1.0	mmol/l
Creatine phosphokinase (CPK)	mU/ml	0.01667	μmol S^{-1}/l
Creatinine	mg/100 ml	88.40	μmol/l
Glucose	mg/100 ml	0.05551	mmol/l
Lactic dehydrogenase	mU/ml	0.01667	μmol S^{-1}/l
Cholesterol	mg/100 ml	0.02586	mmol/l
Magnesium	mEq/l	0.50	mmol/l
P_{CO_2}	mmHg	0.1333	kPa
pH		1.0	l
P_{O_2}	mmHg	0.133	kPa
Phosphatase, acid	Sigma	278.4	nmol S^{-1}/l
Phosphatase, alkaline	Bodansky	0.08967	nmol S^{-1}/l
Phosphorus, inorganic	mg/100 ml	0.3229	mmol/l
Protein, total	g/100 ml	10	g/l
Protein, electrophoreses			
Albumin	% total	0.01	l
Globulin, α_1	% total	0.01	l
α_2	% total	0.01	l
β	% total	0.01	l
γ	% total	0.01	l
Potassium	mEq/l	1.0	mmol/l
Sodium	mEq/l	1.0	mmol/l
Transaminase (SGOT) (aminotransferase)	Karmen	0.008051	μmol S^{-1}/l
Urea nitrogen	mg/100 ml	0.3569	mmol/l
Uric acid	mg/100 ml	0.65948	mmol/l

Source: From Young, D.S. (1975).[6]

Table 139   Approximate Metric and Apothecary Weight Equivalents

Metric	Apothecary	Metric	Apothecary
1 gram (g)	= 15 grains	0.05g (50 mg)	= $^3/_4$ grain
0.6 g (600 mg)	= 10 grains	0.03 g (30 mg)	= $^1/_2$ grain
0.5 g (500 mg)	= 7$^1/_2$ grains	0.015 g (15 mg)	= $^1/_4$ grain
0.3 g (300 mg)	= 5 grains	0.001 g (1 mg)	= 1/80 grain
0.2 g (200 mg)	= 3 grains	0.6 mg	= 1/100 grain
0.1 g (100 mg)	= 1$^1/_2$ grains	0.5 mg	= 1/120 grain
0.06 g (60 mg)	= 1 grain	0.4 mg	= 1/150 grain

Approximate Household, Apothecary, and Metric Volume Equivalents

Household	Apothecary	Metric
1 teaspoon (t or tsp)	= 1 fluidram (f$_3$)	= 4 or 5 ml[a]
1 tablespoon (T or tbs)	= $^1/_2$ fluid ounce (f$_3$)	= 15 ml
2 tablespoons	= 1 fluid ounce	= 30 ml
1 measuring cupful	= 8 fluid ounces	= 240 ml
1 pint (pt)	= 16 fluid ounces	= 473 ml
1 quart (qt)	= 32 fluid ounces	= 946 ml
1 gallon (gal)	= 128 fluid ounces	= 3785 ml

[a] 1 ml = 1 cubic centimeter (cc); however, ml is the preferred measurement term today.

Source: From Beyer, W.H. (1991)[5].

Table 140   Conversion Factors: Metric to English

To Obtain	Multiply	By
Inches	Centimeters	0.3937007874
Feet	Meters	3.280839895
Yards	Meters	1.093613298
Miles	Kilometers	0.6213711922
Ounces	Grams	$3.527396195 \times 10^{-2}$
Pounds	Kilograms	2.204622622
Gallons (U.S. Liquid)	Liters	0.2641720524
Fluid ounces	Milliliters (cc)	$3.381402270 \times 10^{-2}$
Square inches	Square centimeters	0.1550003100
Square feet	Square meters	10.76391042
Square yards	Square meters	1.195990046
Cubic inches	Milliliters (cc)	$6.102374409 \times 10^{-2}$
Cubic feet	Cubic meters	35.31466672
Cubic yards	Cubic meters	1.307950619

Source: From Beyer, W.H. (1991)[5].

Table 141   Conversion Factors: English to Metric

To Obtain	Multiply	By
Microns	Mils	**25.4**
Centimeters	Inches	**2.54**
Meters	Feet	**0.3048**
Meters	Yards	**0.9144**
Kilometers	Miles	**1.609344**
Grams	Ounces	28.34952313
Kilograms	Pounds	**0.45359237**
Liters	Gallons (U.S. Liquid)	**3.785411784**
Millimeters (cc)	Fluid ounces	29.57352956
Square centimeters	Square inches	**6.4516**
Square meters	Square feet	**0.09290304**
Square meters	Square yards	**0.83612736**
Milliliters (cc)	Cubic inches	**16.387064**
Cubic meters	Cubic feet	$2.831684659 \times 10^{-2}$
Cubic meters	Cubic yards	0.764554858

Note: Boldface numbers are exact; others are given to ten significant figures where so indicated by the multiplier factor.

Source: From Beyer, W.H. (1991)[5].

Table 142 Temperature Conversion Factors

°F = 9/5 (°C) + 32

Fahrenheit temperatures = 1.8 (temperature in kelvins) − 459.67

°C = 5/9 [(°F) − 32)]

Celsius temperature = temperature in kelvins − 273.15

Fahrenheit temperature = 1.8 (Celsius temperature) + 32

	Conversion of Temperatures	
From	**To**	
°Celsius	°Fahrenheit	$t_F = (t_C \times 1.8) + 32$
	Kelvin	$T_K = t_C + 273.15$
	°Rankine	$T_R = (t_C + 273.15) \times 18$
°Fahrenheit	°Celsius	$t_C = \dfrac{t_F - 32}{1.8}$
	Kelvin	$T_K = \dfrac{t_F - 32}{1.8} + 273.15$
	°Rankine	$T_R = t_F + 459.67$
Kelvin	°Celsius	$t_C = T_K - 273.15$
	°Rankine	$T_R = T_K \times 1.8$
°Rankine	°Fahrenheit	$t_F = T_R - 459.67$
	Kelvin	$T_K = \dfrac{T_R}{1.8}$

Source: From Beyer, W.H. (1991)[5]; Lide, D.R. (1992)[7].

Table 143 Table of Equivalents

kg	=	1000 g, 1 million mg, 2.2 lb
g	=	1000 mg, 1 million µg, approx. 0.035 oz.
mg	=	1000 µg, 1 million ng
µg	=	1000 ng
l	=	approx. 1 quart, approx. 33 oz.
lb	=	16 oz., 454.5 g, 0.45 kg
oz.	=	28.4 g
acre	=	4047 m²
hectare	=	2.5 acres

When referring to the concentration of a chemical in food or other medium:

mg/kg	=	ppm, µg/g
mg/l	=	ppm = 0.0001%
µg/kg	=	ppb, ng/g
ng/kg	=	ppt
ppm	=	mg/kg, µg/g
ppb	=	µg/kg, ng/g
ppt	=	ng/kg

Source: From Beyer, W.H. (1991)[5]; Lide, D.R. (1992)[7].

Table 144   Standard Atomic Weights

(Scaled to $A_r(^{12}C) = 12$)

The atomic weights of many elements are not invariant but depend on the origin and treatment of the material. The footnotes to this table elaborate the types of variation to be expected for individual elements. The values of $A_r(E)$ and uncertainty $U_r(E)$ given here apply to elements as they exist naturally on earth.

Name	Sym.	Atomic Number	Atomic Weight	Footnotes			
Actinium*	Ac	89					A
Aluminium	Al	13	26.981539(5)				
Americium*	Am	95					A
Antimony (Stibium)	Sb	51	121.75(3)				
Argon	Ar	18	39.948(1)	g		r	
Arsenic	As	33	74.92159(2)				
Astatine*	At	85					A
Barium	Ba	56	137.327(7)				
Berkelium*	Bk	97					A
Beryllium	Be	4	9.012182(3)				
Bismuth	Bi	83	208.98037(3)				
Boron	B	5	10.811(5)	g	m	r	
Bromine	Br	35	79.904(1)				
Cadmium	Cd	48	112.411(8)	g			
Cesium	Cs	55	132.90543(5)				
Calcium	Ca	20	40.078(4)	g			
Californium*	Cf	98					A
Carbon	C	6	12.011(1)			r	
Cerium	Ce	58	140.115(4)	g			
Chlorine	Cl	17	35.4527(9)				
Chromium	Cr	24	51.9961(6)				
Cobalt	Co	27	58.93320(1)				
Copper	Cu	29	63.546(3)			r	
Curium*	Cm	96					A
Dysprosium	Dy	66	162.50(3)	g			
Einsteinium*	Es	99					A
Erbium	Er	68	167.26(3)	g			
Europium	Eu	63	151.965(9)	g			
Fermium*	Fm	100					A

Table 144   Standard Atomic Weights (Continued)

Name	Sym.	Atomic Number	Atomic Weight	Footnotes		
Fluorine	F	9	18.9984032(9)			
Francium*	Fr	87				A
Gadolinium	Gd	64	157.25(3)	g		
Gallium	Ga	31	69.723(1)			
Germanium	Ge	32	72.61(2)			
Gold	Au	79	196.96654(3)			
Hafnium	Hf	72	178.49(2)			
Helium	He	2	4.002602(2)	g	r	
Holmium	Ho	67	164.93032(3)			
Hydrogen	H	1	1.00794(7)	g	m	r
Indium	In	49	114.82(1)			
Iodine	I	53	126.90447(3)			
Iridium	Ir	77	192.22(3)			
Iron	Fe	26	55.847(3)			
Krypton	Kr	36	83.80(1)	g	m	
Lanthanum	La	57	138.9055(2)	g		
Lawrencium*	Lr	103				A
Lead	Pb	82	207.2(1)	g	r	
Lithium	Li	3	6.941(2)	g	m	r
Lutetium	Lu	71	174.967(1)	g		
Magnesium	Mg	12	24.3050(6)			
Manganese	Mn	25	54.93805(1)			
Mendelevium*	Md	101				A
Mercury	Hg	80	200.59(3)			
Molybdenum	Mo	42	95.94(1)			
Neodymium	Nd	60	144.24(3)	g		
Neon	Ne	10	20.1797(6)	g	m	
Neptunium*	Np	93				A
Nickel	Ni	28	58.69(1)			
Niobium	Nb	41	92.90638(2)			
Nitrogen	N	7	14.00674(7)	g	r	
Nobelium*	No	102				A
Osmium	Os	76	190.2(1)	g		
Oxygen	O	8	15.9994(3)	g	r	
Palladium	Pd	46	105.42(1)	g		
Phosphorus	P	15	30.973762(4)			

Table 144 Standard Atomic Weights (Continued)

Name	Sym.	Atomic Number	Atomic Weight		Footnotes
Platinum	Pt	78	195.08(3)		
Plutonium*	Pu	94			A
Polonium*	Po	84			A
Potassium (Kalium)	K	19	39.0983(1)		
Praseodymium	Pr	59	140.90765(3)		
Promethium*	Pm	61			A
Protactinium*	Pa	91			
Radium*	Ra	88			A
Radon*	Rn	86			A
Rhenium	Re	75	186.207(1)		
Rhodium	Rh	45	102.90550(3)		
Rubidium	Rb	37	85.4678(3)	g	
Ruthenium	Ru	44	101.07(2)	g	
Samarium	Sm	62	150.36(3)	g	
Scandium	Sc	21	44.955910(9)		
Selenium	Se	34	78.96(3)		
Silicon	Si	14	28.0855(3)		r
Silver	Ag	47	107.8682(2)	g	
Sodium (Natrium)	Na	11	22.989768(6)		
Strontium	Sr	38	87.62(1)	g	r
Sulfur	S	16	32.066(6)		r
Tantalum	Ta	73	180.9479(1)		
Technetium*	Tc	43			A
Tellurium	Te	52	127.60(3)	g	
Terbium	Tb	65	158.92534(3)		
Thallium	Tl	81	204.3833(2)		
Thorium*	Th	90	232.038(1)	g	Z
Thulium	Tm	69	168.93421(3)		
Tin	Sn	50	118.710(7)	g	
Titanium	Ti	22	47.88(3)		
Tungsten (Wolfram)	W	74	183.85(3)		
Unnilquadium	Unq	104			A
Unnilpentium	Unp	105			A
Unnihexium	Unh	106			A

Table 144   Standard Atomic Weights (Continued)

Name	Sym.	Atomic Number	Atomic Weight		Footnotes	
Unnilseptium	Uns	107				A
Uranium*	U	92	238.0289(1)	g	m	Z
Vanadium	V	23	50.9415(1)			
Xenon	Xe	54	131.29(2)	g	m	
Ytterbium	Yb	70	173.04(3)	g		
Yttrium	Y	39	88.90585(2)			
Zinc	Zn	30	65.39(2)			
Zirconium	Zr	40	91.224(2)	g		

g = Geological specimens are known in which the element has an isotopic composition outside the limits for normal material. The difference between the atomic weight of the element in such specimens and that given in the table may exceed the implied uncertainty.

m = Modified isotopic compositions may be found in commercially available material because it has been subjected to an undisclosed or inadvertent isotopic separation. Substantial deviations in atomic weight of the element from that given in the table can occur.

r = Range in isotopic composition of normal terrestrial material prevents a more precise $A_r(E)$ being given: the tabulated $A_r(E)$ value should be applicable to any normal material.

A = Radioactive element that lacks a characteristic terrestrial isotopic composition.

Z = An element, without stable nuclide(s), exhibiting a range of trial compositions of long-lived radionuclide(s) such that a meaningful atomic weight can be given.

* Element has no stable nuclides.

Source: From Pankow, J.F. (1991)[8].

Table 145 Transformation of Percentages into Logits

Percentage	0	1	2	3	4	5	6	7	8	9
50	0	0.04	0.08	0.12	0.16	0.20	0.24	0.28	0.32	0.36
60	0.41	0.45	0.49	0.53	0.58	0.62	0.66	0.71	0.75	0.80
70	0.85	0.90	0.94	0.99	1.05	1.10	1.15	1.21	1.27	1.32
80	1.38	1.45	1.52	1.59	1.66	1.73	1.82	1.90	1.99	2.09
90	2.20	2.31	2.44	2.59	2.75	2.94	3.18	3.48	3.89	4.60
99	4.60	4.70	4.82	4.95	5.11	5.29	5.52	5.81	6.21	6.91

Source: From Tallarida, R.J. (1992)[9].

Table 146 Transformation of Percentages into Probits

Percentage	0	1	2	3	4	5	6	7	8	9
0	[—]	2.67	2.95	3.12	3.25	3.36	3.45	3.52	3.59	3.66
10	3.72	3.77	3.82	3.87	3.92	3.96	4.01	4.05	4.08	4.12
20	4.16	4.19	4.23	4.26	4.29	4.33	4.36	4.39	4.42	4.45
30	4.48	4.50	4.53	4.56	4.59	4.61	4.64	4.67	4.69	4.72
40	4.75	4.77	4.80	4.82	4.85	4.87	4.90	4.92	4.95	4.97
50	5.00	5.03	5.05	5.08	5.10	5.13	5.15	5.18	5.20	5.23
60	5.25	5.28	5.31	5.33	5.36	5.39	5.41	5.44	5.47	5.50
70	5.52	5.55	5.58	5.61	5.64	5.67	5.71	5.74	5.77	5.81
80	5.84	5.88	5.92	5.95	5.99	6.04	6.08	6.13	6.18	6.23
90	6.28	6.34	6.41	6.48	6.55	6.64	6.75	6.88	7.05	7.33
99	7.33	7.37	7.41	7.46	7.51	7.58	7.65	7.75	7.88	8.07

Source: From Tallarida, R.J. (1992)[9].

Table 147 Molarity, Molality, Normality, Osmolarity Calculations

1. Molarity (M) = $\dfrac{\text{Number of moles of solute}}{\text{Liter of solution}}$

    Where: Number of moles = $\dfrac{\text{Grams of chemical}}{\text{Molecular weight}}$

2. Molality (m) = $\dfrac{\text{Number of moles of solute}}{\text{Kilogram of solution}}$

3. Normality (N) = $\dfrac{\text{Number of equivalents of solute}}{\text{Liter of solution}}$

    Where: Number of equivalents = $\dfrac{\text{Grams of chemical}}{\text{Equivalent weight}}$

    Equivalent weight = $\dfrac{\text{Molecular weight}}{n}$

    For acids and basis, n = The number of replaceable H^+ or OH^- ions per molecule

4. Normality = n Molarity
    Where: n = Number of replaceable H^+ or OH^- ions per molecule

5. Osmolarity = n Molarity
    Where: n = Number of dissociable ions per molecule

Table 148   Solutions Calculations

1. Volume percent (% v/v) $= \dfrac{\text{Volume of solute}}{\text{Volume of solution}} \times 100$

2. Weight percent (% w/w) $= \dfrac{\text{Weight of solute}}{\text{Weight of solution}} \times 100$

3. Weight/volume percent (% w/v) $= \dfrac{\text{Weight of solute (g)}}{\text{Volume of solution (ml)}} \times 100$

4. Milligram percent (mg%) $= \dfrac{\text{Weight of solute (mg)}}{100 \text{ mL of solution}} \times 100$

5. Parts per million (ppm) $= \dfrac{\text{Weight of solute}}{\text{Weight of solution}} \times 10^6$

6. Parts per million (for gasses)

    $$\text{ppm} = \dfrac{(\text{mg/m}^3)(R)}{\text{Molecular weight}}$$

    Where: R = 24.5 at 25°C.

7. $(\text{volume}_C)(\text{concentration}_C) = \text{volume}_D(\text{concentration}_D)$

    Where: C = Concentrated solution

    D = Dilute solution

The above relationship is useful in preparing dilute solutions from concentrated solutions.

Table 149   pH Calculations

1. $\text{pH} = -\log [H^+] = \log \dfrac{1}{[H+]}$

2. $\text{pH} = \text{pKa} + \log \dfrac{[A^-]}{[HA]}$

    Where: HA $\leftrightarrow$ H$^+$ + A$^-$

    (weak acid)   (conjugate base)

    $\text{pK}_a = -\log \text{Ka}$

    (equilibrium constant)

Table 150 Mammalian Toxicology Tests: Cost and Material Requirements

Study Type	Estimated Costs[a]	Estimated Material Requirements[b]
Acute oral toxicity in rats limit test[c]	$500–4500	50 g
Acute oral toxicity in rats, LD_{50} (4 Levels)[d]	$2000–9000	50 g
Acute dermal toxicity in rabbits limit test[c]	$2000–5500	50 g
Acute dermal toxicity in rabbits LD_{50} (4 Levels)[d]	$5500–13,500	100 g
Acute inhalation toxicity in rats (4-hr. exp.) Limit Tests[e]	$4000–12,000	100–5000 g
Acute inhalation toxicity in rats (4-hr. exp.) LC_{50} (4 Levels)[d,e]	$12,000–21,000	500–50,000 g
Primary eye irritation in rabbits[f]	$1000–3000	10 g
Primary skin irritation in rabbits[f]	$1000–2500	10 g
Dermal sensitization in guinea pigs, maximization[g]	$4000–8500	80 g
Dermal sensitization in guinea pigs, Buehler type[g,h]	$4000–7,200	80 g
1-Month oral toxicity in rats-gavage	$44,000–51,000	100–200 g
1-Month inhalation in rats	$100,000–130,000	1–200 kg
1-Month intravenous toxicity in rats	$50,000–60,000	110 150 g
1-Month intravenous toxicity in dogs	$80,000–90,000	2–3 kg
1-Month dermal toxicity in rats	$35,000–50,000	100–300 g
1-Month oral toxicity in dogs-capsule	$75,000–90,000	2–3 kg
3-Month oral toxicity in rats-gavage	$80,000–95,000	600–1200 g
3-Month inhalation in rats[e]	$160,000–220,000	3–600 kg
3-Month inhalation in primate[e]	$250,000–300,000	3–600 kg
3-Month dermal toxicity in rats	$80,000–110,000	300–900 g
3-Month oral toxicity in dogs-capsule	$115,000–130,000	7–10 kg
1-Year oral toxicity in rats-gavage	$200,000–300,000	6–12 kg
1-Year oral toxicity in dogs-capsule	$300,000–400,000	30–40 kg
18-Month oncogenicity in mice-gavage	$500,000–600,000	1–2 kg
24-Month oncogenicity in rats-gavage	$600,000–700,000	12–24 kg
24-Month inhalation in rats[e]	$1,000,000–1,400,000	20–4000 kg
1-Month dietary study in rats	$35,000–45,000	150–200 g
3-Month dietary study in dogs	$110,000–125,000	12–16 kg
24-Month dietary study in rats	$700,000–900,000	16–24 kg
24-Month dietary study in dogs	$300,000–350,000	100–125 kg

Table 150 Mammalian Toxicology Tests: Cost and Material Requirements (Continued)

Study Type	Estimated Costs[a]	Estimated Material Requirements[b]
General fertility and reproductive performance (Segment I) in rats	$95,000–165,000	500–2000 g
Range finding teratology study in rats	$15,000–22,000	50–100 g
Teratology (Segment II) study in rats	$38,000–44,000	50–500 g
Range finding teratology study in rabbits	$29,000–25,000	100–500 g
Teratology (Segment II) study in rabbits	$45,000–52,000	100–1000 g
Perinatal and postnatal study (Segment III) in rats	$60,000–90,000	100–750 g
2-Generation reproduction study in rats	$400,000–800,000	3–12 kg
Human repeat insult patch test (RIPT), 100 subjects, nondedicated panel[i]	$2500 per sample	300–400 g
Human RIPT, 200 subjects, nondedicated panel[i]	$4800 per sample	600–800 g
Human RIPT, 100 subjects, dedicated panel[j]	$24,000 (max. 8–12 samples)	300–400 g

[a] Based on 1993 estimates. Costs, especially for acute studies, can vary widely depending on the endpoints evaluated.

[b] Test sample requirements, especially for longer-term studies by inhalation, can vary considerably and depend on the toxic potency of the test material as well as its physical properties.

[c] Lower cost design may not include control groups, bodyweight measurements, or gross necropsy.

[d] Costs may be higher, depending on histopathology and performance of dose range finding study.

[e] Costs will be higher if analytical method development and/or extraordinary analytical methods required.

[f] Additional cost if extended observation periods required.

[g] Additional cost for positive control.

[h] Number of induction times may vary

[i] Panel may be shared with other sponsors (8–12 samples per subject).

[j] Panel dedicated to one sponsor.

Table 151 Genetic Toxicology Tests: Cost and Material Requirements

Study Type	Estimated Costs[a]	Estimated Material Requirements
Ames assay[b,c]	$2,000–3,000	20 g
Mouse lymphoma assay	$8,000–12,000	5–10 g
In vitro chromosome aberrations (CHO cells)	$7,000–9,000	5 g
In vitro chromosome aberrations (human lymphocytes)	$9,000–13,000	5 g
In vitro chromosome aberrations (rat lymphocytes)	$20,000	5 g
In vivo chromosome aberrations (mouse bone marrow)	$24,000–28,000	25–50 g
In vivo chromosome aberration (rat bone marrow)	$30,000	50–100 g
In vitro Unscheduled DNA Synthesis (UDS)	$7,000–8,000	5 g
In vivo/In vitro UDS	$20,000–26,000	25–50 g
In vitro cell transformation (Syrian Hamsters)	$13,000–16,000	5 g
Drosophilia sex-linked recessive lethal	$30,000–35,000	50 g
Dominant Lethal (Mouse)	$25,000	25–50 g
Dominant Lethal (Rat)	$28,000	100 g

[a] Costs will be higher if confirmatory studies required. Costs based on 1993 estimates.

[b] Costs will vary, depending on method of liver enzyme exposure.

[c] Costs will be higher if additional bacterial strains required.

Table 152   Aquatic/Ecotoxicology Tests: Cost and Material Requirements

Study Type	Estimated Cost[a]	Estimated Material Requirements
Fish static acute (freshwater) (96 hr)[b]	$3,000	10 g
Fish 35-day embryo/larval	$25,000	150 g[c]
Fish 90-day embryo/larval	$37,000	350 g[c]
Daphnid static acute (48 hr)[b]	$2,900	5 g
Daphnid 21-day chronic reproduction	$19,500	100 g[c]
Algal static acute[b] (96 hr)	$4,500	5 g
Algal static 14-day[b]	$6,700	5 g
28-Day bioconcentration with depuration phase	$34,500	200 g[c]
Earthworm (48 hr —filter paper)	$3,500	5 g
Earthworm (114 day–soil)	$4,500	30 g

[a]   Costs will be higher if analytical method development and/or extraordinary analytic methods are required. Costs based on 1993 estimates.

[b]   Additional cost if flow-through design required.

[c]   Assumes highest test concentration of 10 mg/L.

Table 153   Chemical Functional Groups

Acetamido (acetylamino)	CH_3CONH-
Acetimido (acetylimino)	$CH_3C(=NH)-$
Acetoacetamido	CH_3COCH_2CONH-
Acetoacetyl	CH_3COCH_2CO-
Acetonyl	CH_3COCH_2
Acetonylidene	$CH_3COCH=$
Acetyl	CH_3CO-
Acrylyl	$CH_2=CHCO-$
Adipyl (from adipic acid)	$-OC(CH_2)_4CO-$
Alanyl (from alanine)	$CH_3CH(NH_2)CO-$
β-Alanyl	$H\ N(CH_2)_2CO-$
Allophanoyl	$H_2NCONHCO-$
Allyl (2-propenyl)	$CH_2=CHCH_2-$
Allylidene (2-propenylidene)	$CH_2=CHCH=$

Table 153　Chemical Functional Groups (Continued)

Amidino (aminoiminomethyl)	$H_2NC(=NH)-$
Amino	H_2N-
Amyl (pentyl)	$CH_3(CH_2)_4-$
Anilino (phenylamino)	C_6H_5NH-
Anisidino	$CH_3OC_6H_4NH-$
Anisyl (from anisic acid)	$CH_3OC_6H_4CO-$
Anthranoyl (2-aminobenzoyl)	$2-H_2NC_6H_4CO-$
Arsino	AsH_2-
Azelaoyl (from azelaic acid)	$-OC(CH_2)_7CO-$
Azido	$N_3=$
Azino	$=NN=$
Azo	$-N=N-$
Azoxy	$-N(O)N-$
Benzal	$C_6H_5CH=$
Benzamido (benzylamino)	C_6H_5CONH-
Benzhydryl (diphenylmethyl)	$(C_6H_5)_2CH-$
Benzimido (benzylimino)	$C_6H_5C(=NH)-$
Benzoxy (benzoyloxy)	C_6H_5COO-
Benzoyl	C_6H_5CO-
Benzyl	$C_6H_5CH_2-$
Benzylidine	$C_6H_5CH=$
Benzyldyne	$C_6H_5C\equiv$
Biphenylyl	$C_6H_5C_6H_5-$
Biphenylene	$-C_6H_4C_6H_4-$
Butoxy	C_4H_9O-
sec-Butoxy	$C_2H_5CH(CH_3)O-$
tert-Butoxy	$(CH_3)_3CO-$
Butyl	$CH_3(CH_2)_3-$
iso-Butyl (3-methylpropyl)	$(CH_3)_2(CH_2)_2-$
sec-Butyl (1-methylpropyl)	$C_2H_5CH(CH_3)-$
tert-Butyl (1,1, dimethylethyl)	$(CH_3)_3C-$
Butyryl	C_3H_7CO-
Caproyl (from caproic acid)	$CH_3(CH_2)_4CO-$
Capryl (from capric acid)	$CH_3(CH_2)_6CO-$
Caprylyl (from caprylic acid)	$CH_3(CH_2)_6CO-$
Carbamido	$H_2NCONH-$

Table 153   Chemical Functional Groups (Continued)

Carbamoyl (aminocarbonyl)	H_2NCO-
Carbamyl (aminocarbonyl)	H_2NCO-
Carbazoyl (hydrazinocarbonyl)	$H_2NNHCO-$
Carbethoxy	$C_2H_5O_2C-$
Carbobenzoxy	$C_6H_5CH_2O_2C-$
Carbonyl	$-C=O-$
Carboxy	$HOOC-$
Cetyl	$CH_3(CH_2)_{15}-$
Chloroformyl (chlorocarbonyl)	$CLCO-$
Cinnamyl (3-phenyl-2-propenyl)	$C_6H_5CH=CHCH_2-$
Cinnamoyl	$C_6H_5CH=CHCO-$
Cinnamylidene	$C_6H_5CH=CHCH=$
Cresyl (hydroxymethylphenyl)	$HO(CH_3)C_6H_4-$
Crotoxyl	$CH_3CH=CHCO-$
Crotoyl (2-butenyl)	$CH_3CH=CHCH_2$
Cyanamido (cyanoamino)	$NCNH-$
Cyanato	$NCO-$
Cyano	$NC-$
Decanedioyl	$-OC(CH_2)_6CO-$
Decanoly	$CH_3(CH_2)_6CO-$
Diazo	$N_2=$
Diazoamino	$-NHN=N-$
Disilanyl	H_2SiSiH_2-
Disiloxanoxy	$H_3SiOSiH_2O)-$
Disulfinyl	$-S(O)S(O)-$
Dithio	$-SS-$
Enanthyl	$CH_3(CH_2)_5CO-$
Epoxy	$-O-$
Ethenyl (vinyl)	$CH_2=CH-$
Ethinyl	$HC\equiv C-$
Ethoxy	C_2H_5O-
Ethyl	CH_3CH_2-
Ethylthio	C_2H_5S
Formamido (formylamino)	$HCONH-$
Formyl	$HCO-$

Table 153 Chemical Functional Groups (Continued)

Fumaroyl (from fumaric acid)	$-OCCH=CHCO-$
Furfuryl (2-furanylmethyl)	$OC_4H_3CH_2-$
Furfurylidene (2-furanylmethylene)	$OC_4H_3CH=$
Furyl (furanyl)	OC_4H_3-
Glutamyl (from glutamic acid)	$-OC(CH_2)_2CH(NH_2)CO-$
Glutaryl (from glutaric acid)	$-OC(CH_2)CO-$
Glycidyl (oxiranylmethyl)	CH_2-CHCH_2-
Glycinamido	H_2NCH_2CONH-
Glycolyl (hydroxyacetyl)	$HOCH_2CO-$
Glycyl (aminoacetyl)	H_2NCH_2CO-
Glyoxylyl (oxoacetyl)	$HCOCO-$
Guanidino	$H_2NC(=NH)NH-$
Guanyl	$H_2NC(=NH)-$
Heptadecanoyl	$CH_3(CH_2)_{15}CO-$
Heptanamido	$CH_3(CH_2)_{15}CONH-$
Heptanedioyl	$-OC(CH_2)_5CO-$
Heptanoyl	$CH_3(CH_2)_5CO-$
Hexadecanoyl	$CH_3(CH_2)_4CO-$
Hexamethylene	$-(CH_2)_6-$
Hexanedioyl	$-OC(CH_2)_4CO-$
Hippuryl (N-benzoylglycyl)	$C_6H_5CONHCH_2CO-$
Hydantoyl	$H_2NCONHCH_2CO-$
Hydrazino	N_2NNH-
Hydrazo	$-HNNH-$
Hydrocinnamoyl	$C_6H_5(CH_2)_2CO-$
Hydroperoxy	$HOO-$
Hydroxamino	$HONH-$
Hydroxy	$HO-$
Imino	$HN=$
Iodoso	$OI-$
Isoamyl (isopentyl)	$(CH_3)_2CH(CH_2)_2-$
Isobutenyl (2-methyl-1-propenyl)	$(CH_3)_2C=CH-$
Isobutoxy	$(CH_3)_2CHCHO-$
Isobutyl	$(CH_3)_2CHCH_2-$
Isobutylidene	$(CH_3)_2CHCH=$

Table 153   Chemical Functional Groups (Continued)

Isobutyryl	$(CH_3)_2CHCO-$
Isocyanato	$OCN-$
Isocyano	$CN-$
Isohexyl	$(CH_3)_2CH(CH_2)_3-$
Isoleucyl (from isoleucine)	$C_2H_3CH(CH_3)CH(NH_4)CO-$
Isonitroso	$HON=$
Isopentyl	$(CH_3)_2CH(CH_2)_2-$
Isopentylidene	$(CH_3)_2CHCH_2CH=$
Isopropenyl	$H_2C=C(CH_3)-$
Isopropoxy	$(CH_3)_2CHO-$
Isopropyl	$(CH_3)_2CH-$
Isopropylidene	$(CH_3)_2C=$
Isothiocyanato (isothiocyano)	$SCN-$
Isovaleryl (from isovaleric acid)	$(CH_3)_2CHCH_2CO-$
Keto (oxo)	$O=$
Lactyl (from lactic acid)	$CH_3CH(OH)CO-$
Lauroyl (from lauric acid)	$CH_3(CH_2)_{10}CO-$
Laucyl (from leucine)	$(CH_3)_2CHCH_2CH(NH_2)CO-$
Levulinyl (from levulinic acid)	$CH_3CO(CH_2)_2CO-$
Malonyl (from malonic acid)	$-OCCH_2CO-$
Mandelyl (from mandelic acid	$C_6H_5CH(OH)CO-$
Mercapto	$HS-$
Methacrylyl (from methacrylic acid)	$CH_2=C(CH_3)CO-$
Methallyl	$CH_2=C(CH_3)CH_2-$
Methionyl (from methionine)	$CH_3SCH_2CH_2CH(NH_2)CO-$
Methoxy	CH_3O-
Methyl	H_3C-
Methylene	$H_2C=$
Methylenedioxy	$-OCH_2O-$
Methylenedisulfonyl	$-O_2SCH_2SO_2-$
Methylol	$HOCH_2-$
Methylthio	CH_2S-
Myristyl (from myristic acid)	$CH_3(CH_2)_{12}CO-$
Naphthal	$(C_{10}H_7)CH=$
Naphthobenzyl	$(C_{10}H_7)CH_2-$

Table 153   Chemical Functional Groups (Continued)

Naphthoxy	$(C_{10}H_7)O-$
Naphthyl	$(C_{10}H_7)-$
Naphthylidene	$(C_{10}H_6)=$
Neopentyl	$(CH_3)_3CCH_2-$
Nitramino	O_2NNH-
Nitro	O_2N-
Nitrosamino	$ONNH-$
Nitrosimino	$ONN=$
Nitroso	$ON-$
Nonanoyl (from nonanoic acid)	$CH_3(CH_2)_7CO-$
Oleyl (from oleic acid)	$CH_3(CH_2)_7CH=CH(CH_2)_7CO-$
Oxalyl (from oxalic acid)	$-OCCO-$
Oxamido	$H_2NCOCONH-$
Oxo (keto)	$O=$
Palmityl (from palmitic acid)	$CH_3(CH_2)_{14}CO-$
Pelargonyl (from pelargonic acid)	$CH_3(CH_2)_7CO-$
Pentamethylene	$-(CH_2)_5-$
Pentyl	$CH_3(CH_2)_4-$
Phenacyl	$C_6H_5COCH_2-$
Phenacylidene	$C_6H_5COCH=$
Phenanthryl	$(C_{14}H_9)-$
Phenethyl	$C_6H_5CH_2CH_2-$
Phenoxy	C_6H_5O-
Phenyl	C_6H_5-
Phenylene	$-C_6H_4-$
Phenylenedioxy	$-OC_6H_4O-$
Phosphino	H_2P-
Phosphinyl	$H_2P(O)-$
Phospho	O_2P-
Phosphono	$(HO)_2P(O)-$
Phthalyl (from phthalic acid)	$1,2-C_6H_4(CO-)_2$
Picryl (2,4,6-trinitrophenyl)	$2,4,6-(NO_2)_2C_6H_2-$
Pimelyl (from pimelic acid)	$-OC(CH_2)_5CO-$
Piperidino	$C_5H_{10}N-$
Piperidyl (piperidinyl)	$(C_5H_{10}N)-$
Piperonyl	$3,4-(CH_2O_2)C_6H_3CH_2-$
Pivalyl (from pivalic acid)	$(CH_3)_3CCO-$
Prenyl (3-methyl-2-butenyl)	$(CH_3)_2C=CHCH_2-$
Propargyl (2-propynyl)	$HC\equiv CCH_2-$

Table 153   Chemical Functional Groups (Continued)

Propenyl	$CH_2=CHCH_2-$
iso-Propenyl	$(CH_3)_2C=$
Propionyl	CH_3CH_2CO-
Propoxy	$CH_3CH_2CH_2O-$
Propyl	$CH_3CH_2CH_2-$
iso-Propyl	$(CH_3)_2CH-$
Propylidene	$CH_3CH_2CH=$
Pyridino	C_5H_5N-
Pyridyl (pyridinyl)	$(C_5H_4N)-$
Pyrryl (pyrrolyl)	$(C_3H_4N)-$
Salicyl (2-hydroxybenzoyl)	$2\text{-}HOC_6H_4CO-$
Selenyl	$HSe-$
Seryl (from serine)	$HOCH_2CH(NH_2)CO-$
Siloxy	H_3SiO-
Silyl	H_3Si-
Silylene	$H_2Si=$
Sorbyl (from sorbic acid)	$CH_3CH=CHCH=CHCO-$
Stearyl (from stearic acid)	$CH_3(CH_2)_{16}CO-$
Styryl	$C_6H_5CH=CH-$
Suberyl (from suberic acid)	$-OC(CH_2)_6CO-$
Succinamyl	$H_2NCOCH_2CH_2CO-$
Succinyl (from succinic acid)	$-OCCH_2CH_2CO-$
Sulfamino	$HOSO_2NH-$
Sulfamyl	H_2NSO-
Sulfanilyl	$4\text{-}H_2NC_6H_4SO_2-$
Sulfeno	$HOS-$
Sulfhydryl (mercapto)	$HS-$
Sulfinyl	$OS=$
Sulfo	HO_3S-
Sulfonyl	$-SO_2-$
Terephthalyl	$1,4\text{-}C_6H_4(CO-)_2$
Tetramethylene	$-(CH_2)_4-$
Thenyl	$(C_4H_3S)CH-$
Thienyl	$(C_4H_3S)-$
Thiobenzoyl	C_6H_5CS-
Thiocarbamyl	H_2NCS-

Table 153   Chemical Functional Groups (Continued)

Thiocarbonyl	–CS–
Thiocarboxy	HOSC–
Thiocyanato	NCS–
Thionyl (sulfinyl)	–SO–
Thiophenacyl	$C_6H_5CSCH_2$–
Thiuram (aminothioxomethyl)	H_2NCS–
Threonyl (from threonine)	$CH_3CH(OH)CH(NH_2)CO$–
Toluidino	$CH_3C_6H_4NH$–
Toluyl	$CH_3C_6H_4CO$–
Tolyl (methylphenyl)	$CH_3C_6H_4$–
α-Tolyl	$C_6H_5CH_2$–
Tolylene (methylphenylene)	$(CH_3C_6H_3)=$
α-Tolylene	$C_6H_5CH=$
Tosyl [(4-methylphenyl) sulfonyl)]	$4-CH_3C_6H_4SO_2$–
Triazano	H_2NNHNH–
Trimethylene	$-(CH_2)_3$–
Triphenylmethyl (trityl)	$(C_6H_5)_3C$–
Tyrosyl (from tyrosine)	$4-HOC_6H_4CH_2CH(NH_2)CO$–
Ureido	H_2NCONH–
Valeryl (from valeric acid)	C_4H_9CO
Valyl (from valine)	$(CH_3)_2CHCH(NH_2)CO$–
Vinyl	$CH_2=CH$–
Vinylidene	$CH_2=C=$
Xenyl (biphenylyl)	$C_6H_5C_6H_4$–
Xylidino	$(CH_3)_2C_6H_3NH$–
Xylyl (dimethylphenyl)	$(CH_3)_2C_6H_3$–
Xylylene	$-CH_2C_6H_4CH_2$–

Source: From Lide, D.R., Ed. (1992).[6]

References

1. Illing, *Xenobiotic Metabolism and Disposition: The Design of Studies on Novel Compounds*, CRC Press, Boca Raton, FL, 1989.

2. Niesink, R.J.M., deVries, J., and Hollinger, M.A., *Toxicology: Principles and Applications*, CRC Press, Boca Raton, FL, 1996.

3. Mitruka, B.M. and Rawnsley, H.M., *Clinical Biochemical and Hematological Reference Values in Normal Experimental Animals*, Masson Publishing, New York, 1977.

4. Sipes, I.G. and Gandolfi, A.J., in *Casarett and Doull's Toxicology. The Basic Science of Poisons*, 3rd ed., Doull, J., Klaassen, C.D., and Amdur, M.O., Eds., Macmillan, New York, 1992, 88.

5. Beyer, W.H. Ed., *CRC Standard Mathematical Tables and Formulae*, 29th ed., CRC Press, Boca Raton, FL, 1991.

6. Young, D.S., *N. Engl. J. Med.*, 292, 795, 1975.

7. Lide, D.R., Ed., *CRC Handbook of Chemistry and Physics*, 73rd ed., Boca Raton, FL, CRC Press, 1992.

8. Pankow, J.F., *Aquatic Chemistry Concepts*, Lewis Publishers, Chelsea, MI, 1991.

9. Tallarida, R.J., *Pocket Book of Integrals and Mathematical Formulas*, 2nd ed., CRC Press, Boca Raton, FL, 1992.

Section 14:
Glossary

DERMAL TOXICOLOGY

Acanthosis: Hypertrophy of the stratum spinosum and granulosum.

Blanching: To take color from, to bleach. Characterized by a white or pale discoloration of the exposure area due to decreased blood flow to the skin (ischemia).

Contact dermatitis: A delayed type of induced sensitivity (allergy) of the skin with varying degrees of erythema, edema, and vesiculation, resulting from cutaneous contact with a specific allergen.

Contact urticaria: Wheal-and-flare response elicited within 30 to 60 minutes after cutaneous exposure to test substance. May be IgE mediated or non-immunologically mediated.

Corrosion: Direct chemical action on normal living skin that results in its disintegration and irreversible alteration at the site of contact. Corrosion is manifested by ulceration and necrosis with subsequent scar formation.

Cumulative Irritation: Primary irritation resulting from repeated exposures to materials that do not in themselves cause acute primary irritation.

Dermatitis: Inflammation of the skin.

Desquamation: The shedding of the cuticle in scales or the outer layer of any surface. To shred, peel, or scale off, as the casting off of the epidermis in scales or shred, or the shedding of the outer layer of any surface.

Eczema: Inflammatory condition in which the skin becomes red and small vesicles, crusts, and scales develop.

Edema: An excessive accumulation of serious fluid or water in cells, tissues, or serous cavities.

Erythema: An inflammatory redness of the skin, as caused by chemical poisoning or sunburn, usually a result of congestion of the capillaries.

Eschar: A dry scab, thick coagulated crust or slough formed on the skin as a result of a thermal burn or by the action of a corrosive or caustic substance.

Exfoliation: To remove in flakes or scales, peel. To cast off in scales, flakes, or the like. To come off or separate as scales, flakes, sheets, or layers. Detachment and shedding of superficial cells of an epithelium or from any tissue surface. Scaling or desquamation of the horny layer of epidermis, which varies in amount from minute quantities to shedding the entire integument.

Hyperkeratosis: Hypertrophy and thickening of the stratum corneum.

Irritant: A substance that causes inflammation and other evidence of irritation, particularly of the skin, on first contact or exposure; a reaction of irritation not dependent on a mechanism of sensitization.

Irritation: A local reversible inflammatory response of normal living skin to direct injury caused by a single application of a toxic substance, without the involvement of an immunologic mechanism.

Necrosis: Pathological death of one or more cells, or of a portion of tissue or organ, resulting from irreversible damage.

Non-occlusive: Site of application of test substance is open to the air.

Occlusive: A bandage or dressing that covers the skin and excludes it from air. Prevents loss of a test substance by evaporation and by increasing tissue penetration.

Photoallergy: An increased reactivity of the skin to UV and/or visible radiation produced by a chemical agent on an immunologic basis. Previous allergy sensitized by exposure to the chemical agent and appropriate radiation is necessary. The main role of light in photoallergy appears to be in the conversion of the hapten to a complete allergen.

Photoirritation: Irritation resulting from light-induced molecular changes in the structure of chemicals applied to the skin.

Photosensitization: Sensitization of the skin to ultraviolet (UV) light, usually due to the action of certain drugs, plants, or other substances; may occur shortly after administration of the substance, or may occur only after latent period of days to months. The processes whereby foreign substances, either absorbed locally into the skin or systemically, may be subjected to photochemical reactions within the skin, leading to either chemically induced photosensitivity reactions or altering the "normal" pathologic effects of light. UV-A is usually responsible for most photosensitivity reactions.

Semi-occlusive: Site of application of test substance is covered; however, movement of air through covering is not restricted.

Sensitization (allergic contact dermatitis): An immunologically mediated cutaneous reaction to a substance.

Superficial sloughing: Characterized by dead tissue separated from a living structure. Any outer layer or covering that is shed. Necrosed tissue separated from the living structure.

Ulceration: The development of an inflammatory, often suppurating lesion, on the skin or an internal mucous surface of the body caused by superficial loss of tissue, resulting in necrosis of the tissue.

Ocular Toxicology

Anterior chamber: The aqueous-containing cavity of the eye, bounded by the cornea anteriorly, the chamber angle structures peripherally, and the iris and lens posteriorly.

Blepharitis: Inflammation of the eyelids.

Blepharospasm: Involuntary spasm of the eyelids.

Cataract: An opacity of the lens or its capsule.

Chemosis: Intense edema of the conjunctiva. The conjunctiva is loose fibrovascular connective tissue that is relatively rich in lymphatics and responds to noxious stimuli by swelling to the point of prolapse between the eyelids.

Choroid: The vascular middle coat between the retina and sclera.

Ciliary body: The portion of the uveal tract between the iris and the choroid, consisting of ciliary processes and the ciliary muscle.

Conjunctiva: Mucous membrane that lines the posterior aspect of the eyelids (palpebral conjunctiva) and the anterior sclera (bulbar conjunctiva).

Conjunctivitis: Inflammation of the conjunctiva.

Cornea: Transparent portion of the outer coat of the eyeball forming the anterior wall of the anterior chamber.

Exophthalmos: Abnormal protrusion of the eyeball.

Fluorescein (Fluorescein sodium): A fluorescent dye, the simplest of the fluorane dyes and the mother substance of eosin, which is commonly used intravenously to determine the state of adequacy of circulation in the retina and to a lesser degree the chorioid and iris. Another important use is to detect epithelial lesions of the cornea and conjunctiva. Peak excitation occurs with light at a wavelength between 485 and 500 millimicrons, and peak emission occurs between 520 and 530 millimicrons.

Fovea: Depression in the macula adapted for most acute vision.

Fundus: The posterior portion of the eye visible through an ophthalmoscope.

Hyperemia: Excess of blood in a part due to local or general relaxation of the arterioles. Blood vessels become congested and give the area involved a reddish or red-blue color.

Injection: Congestion of blood vessels.

Iris: The circular pigmented membrane behind the cornea and immediately in front of the lens; the most anterior portion of the vascular tunic of the eye. It is composed of the dilator and sphincter muscles, the two-layered posterior epithelium, and mesodermal components that form the iris stroma.

Iritis: Inflammation of the iris, manifested by vascular congestion (hyperemia). An outpouring of serum proteins into the aqueous (flare) may accompany the inflammatory reaction.

Keratitis: Inflammation of the cornea.

Lens: A transparent biconvex structure suspended in the eyeball between the aqueous and the vitreous. Its function is to bring rays of light to focus on the retina. Accommodation is produced by variations in the magnitude of this effect.

Miotic: A drug causing pupillary constriction.

Mydriatic: A drug causing pupillary dilatation.

Nystagmus: An involuntary, rapid movement of the eyeball that may be horizontal, vertical, rotatory, or mixed.

Optic disk: Ophthalmoscopically visible portion of the optic nerve.

Palpebral: Pertaining to the eyelid.

Pannus: Vascularization and connective-tissue deposition beneath the epithelium of the cornea.

Posterior chamber: Space filled with aqueous anterior to the lens and posterior to the iris.

Ptosis: Drooping of the upper eyelid.

Pupil: The round opening at the center of the iris that allows transmission of light to the posterior of the eyeball.

Retina: The innermost or nervous tunic of the eye that is derived from the optic cup (the outer layer develops into the complex sensory layer).

Sclera: The white, tough covering of the eye that, with the cornea, forms the external protective coat of the eye.

Vitreous: Transparent, colorless mass of soft, gelatinous material filling the space in the eyeball posterior to the lens and anterior to the retina.

IMMUNOTOXICOLOGY

ADCC (antibody-dependent cell-mediated cytotoxicity): A specific form of cell-mediated immunity in which an antibody binds a target and a cytotoxic cell (either a macrophage or lymphocyte), linking the two together prior to lysis of the target cell.

Adjuvant: Any material that enhances an immune response, it generally refers to a mixture of oil and mycobacterial cell fragments.

Antibody: Complex molecules produced by plasma cells that recognize specific antigens. Antibodies, also termed immunoglobins (Ig), consist of two basic units. The antigen-binding section (Fab) contains variable regions coding for antigen recognition. The constant region of the molecule (Fc) may be grouped into several classes, designated IgA, IgD, IgE, IgG, and IgM, depending on the molecules' function. Cross-linking of antibody molecules on the surface of a target leads to activation of complement, usually resulting in the destruction of the target.

Antibody-forming cell (AFC)/Plaque-forming cell (PFC) assay: The AFC assay measures the ability of animals to produce either IgM or IgG antibodies against a T-dependent or T-independent antigen following *in vivo* sensitization. Due to the involvement of multiple cell populations in mounting an antibody response, the AFC assay actually evaluates several immune parameters simultaneously. It is considered to be one of the most sensitive indicator systems for immunotoxicology studies.

Antigen: A molecule that is the subject of a specific immune reaction. Antigens are recognized in a cognate fashion by either immunoglobulins or the T-cell antigen receptor. Antigens are often proteinaceous in nature.

Antigen-presenting cell (APC): Cells that are responsible for making antigens accessible to immune effector and regulatory cells. Following internalization and degradation of the antigen (generally by phagocytosis), a fragment of the antigen molecule is presented on the APC cell surface in association with an MHC molecule. This complex is recognized by either B-cells via surface-bound immunoglobulin molecules, or by T-cells via the T-cell antigen receptor. Induction of a specific immune response then proceeds. APC include macrophages, dendritic cells, and certain B-cells.

B-cell/B-lymphocyte: Lymphocytes that recognize antigen via surface-bound immunoglobulins. B-cells that have been exposed to specific antigen differentiate into plasma cells, which are responsible for producing specific antibodies. B-cells differentiate in the bone marrow in mammals, and in an organ known as the bursa in birds.

CD (cluster of differentiation): The CD series is used to denote cell surface markers (e.g., CD4, CD8). These markers, used experimentally as a means of identifying cell types, also serve physiological roles.

CMI (cell-mediated immunity): Antigen-specific immune reactivity mediated primarily by T-lymphocytes. Cell-mediated immunity can be expressed as immune regulatory activity (primarily mediated by CD4+ T-helper cells) or immune effector activity (mediated largely by CD8+ T-cytotoxic cell). Other forms of direct cellular activity (e.g., NK cells, macrophages) are generally not antigen-specific (i.e., non-immune) and are more accurately described as natural immunity.

Complement: A group of approximately 20 proteinase precursors that interact in a cascading fashion. Following activation, the various precursors interact to form a complex that eventually leads to osmotic lysis of a target cell.

Cytokine: Small peptides produced by cells of the immune system (primarily T-helper cells) that subserve a wide range of regulatory and effector mechanisms. Cytokines may be roughly grouped into non-exclusive categories, including interleukins (IL-1–IL-15), tumor necrosis factors, interferons, colony-stimulating factors, and miscellaneous other growth factors.

Cytotoxic T-lymphocyte (CTL): A subset of T-lymphocytes bearing the CD8 surface marker, CTLs are able to kill target cells following induction of a specific immune response. The mechanism of this lysis is controversial, but may result from a combination of direct lysis resulting from extrusion of lytic granules by the CTL, as well as the induction of apoptosis (programmed cell death) in the target cell. The target cells most frequently used for assessment of CTL activity are virally infected cells and tumor cells. Measurement of CTL activity provides an indication of cell-mediated immunity.

Delayed-type hypersensitivity (DTH): A form of cell-mediated immunity in which recall exposure to an antigen results in an inflammatory reaction mediated by T-lymphocytes. Usually expressed as contact hypersensitivity.

ELISA (Enzyme-Linked ImmunoSorbent Assay): A type of immunoassay in which specific antibodies are used to both capture and detect antigens of interest. The most popular type is the "sandwich" ELISA, in which antibodies are bound to a substrate such as a plastic culture plate. These antibodies bind antigenic determinants on molecules (or alternatively on whole cells). Unrelated material is washed away, and the plates are exposed to an antibody of a different specificity; this antibody is coupled to a detector molecule.

Hapten: Low-molecular-weight molecules that are not antigenic by themselves, but are recognized as antigens when bound to larger molecules such as proteins.

HMI (humoral-mediated immunity): Specific immune responses that are mediated primarily by humoral factors (i.e., antibodies and complement). The induction of humoral immune responses generally requires the cooperation of cellular immune mechanisms.

Hybridoma: A genetically engineered cell clone which produced antibodies of a single type (i.e., monoclonal antibodies). Monoclonal antibodies are highly specific for their cognate antigen and make highly useful tools for immunotoxicological studies.

Macrophage: A bone-marrow-derived cell that is present in the peripheral tissue; macrophages found in the circulation are referred to as monocytes. Macrophages serve a wide variety of host defense needs, acting as both non-specific killer cells and as regulators of other immune and non-immune host resistance mechanisms.

MHC (major histocompatibility complex): Murine cell surface molecules for which two major classes are recognized: Class I (present on all nucleated cells) and Class II (present on B-cells, T-cells, and macrophages). MHC molecules appear to direct the course of immune reactivity and are presented in association with antigen by antigen-presenting cells. The human equivalent is termed HLA (human leukocyte antigen).

Mitogen: Mitogens are molecules capable of inducing cellular activation and may include sugars or peptides. The ability of a cell to respond to stimulation with a mitogen (generally assessed by cellular proliferation) is thought to give an indication of the cell's immune responsiveness. Mitogens most commonly employed in immunotoxicology assays include the T-cell mitogens Concanavalin A (ConA) and phytohemagglutinin (PHA). Mitogens routinely used for assessing B-cell proliferation include pokeweed mitogen (PWM) and *E. coli* lipopolysaccharide (LPS).

Natural (nonspecific) immunity: Host defense mechanisms that do not require prior exposure to antigen. The actions of macrophages and NK cells are examples.

Natural killer (NK) cells: A population of lymphocytes separate from T- and B-lymphocytes, also referred to as large granular lymphocytes (LGL). NK cells exhibit cytotoxicity against virally infected cells and certain tumor cells. They are notable in that they do not require prior exposure to antigen to express cytotoxicity toward their targets. Assessment of NK activity provides a measurement of non-specific host resistance.

RES (reticuloendothelial system): The system composed of all phagocytic cells of the body, including monocytes and tissue macrophages. This system is now more commonly known as the Mononuclear Phagocytic System.

T-cell/T-lymphocyte: Lymphocytes that recognize specific antigen via a complex of molecules known as the T-cell antigen receptor (TCR). These cells are primarily responsible for the induction and maintenance of cell-mediated immunity, although they also regulate humoral-mediated immunity and certain non-immune effector mechanisms. A variety of T-cell subtypes have been described, including T-helper cell, T-cytotoxic cells, T-suppressor cells, and T-inducer cells. T-cells mature in the thymus.

Xenobiotic: Any substance that is foreign to the immune system. In the context of immunotoxicology, the term generally refers to non-biological chemicals or drugs.

CARCINOGENESIS*

Adduct: The covalent linkage or addition product between an alkylating agent and cellular macromolecules such as protein, RNA, and DNA.

Alkylating agent: A chemical compound that has positively charged (electron-deficient) groups that can form covalent linkages with negatively charged portions of biological molecules such as DNA. The covalent linkage is referred to as an adduct and may have mutagenic or carcinogenic effects on the organism. The alkyl species is the radical that results when an aliphatic hydrocarbon loses one hydrogen atom to become electron-deficient. Alkylating agents react primarily with guanine, adding their alkyl group to N7 of the purine ring.

---

* Reprinted in part from Maronpot, R.R., *Handbook of Toxicological Pathology*, Academic Press, San Diego, 1991, 127–129. With permission.

Altered focus: A histologically identifiable clone of cells within an organ that differs phenotypically from the normal parenchyma. Foci of altered cells usually result from increased cellular proliferation, represent clonal expansions of initiated cells, and are frequently observed in multistage animal models of carcinogenesis. Foci of cellular alteration are most commonly observed in the liver of carcinogen-treated rodents and are believed by some to represent preneoplastic lesions.

Benign: A classification of anticipated biological behavior of neoplasms in which the prognosis for survival is good. Benign neoplasms grow slowly, remain localized, and usually cause little harm to the patient.

Choristoma: A mass of well-differentiated cells from one organ included within another organ (e.g., adrenal tissue present in the lung).

Chromosomal aberration: A numerical or structural chromosomal abnormality.

Co-carcinogen: An agent not carcinogenic alone but that potentiates the effect of a known carcinogen.

Co-carcinogenesis: The augmentation of neoplasm formation by simultaneous administration of a genotoxic carcinogen and an additional agent (co-carcinogen) that has no inherent carcinogenic activity by itself.

Direct carcinogen: Carcinogens that have the necessary structure to directly interact with cellular constituents and cause neoplasia. Direct-acting carcinogens do not require metabolic conversion by the host to be active. They are considered genotoxic because they typically undergo covalent binding to DNA.

Dysplasia: Disordered tissue formation characterized by changes in size, shape, and orientational relationships of adult types of cells. Primarily seen in epithelial cells.

Epigenetic: Change in phenotype without a change in DNA structure. One of two main mechanisms of carcinogens action, epigenetic carcinogens are nongenotoxic (i.e., they do not form reactive intermediates that interact with genetic material in the process of producing or enhancing neoplasm formation).

Genotoxic carcinogen: An agent that interacts with cellular DNA either directly in its parent form (direct carcinogen) or after metabolic biotransformation.

Hyperplasia: A numerical increase in the number of phenotypically normal cells within a tissue or organ.

Hypertrophy: An increase in the size of an organelle, cell, tissue, or organ within a living organism. To be distinguished from hyperplasia, hypertrophy refers to an increase in size rather than an increase in number. Excessive hyperplasia in a tissue may produce hypertrophy of the organ in which that tissue occurs.

Initiation: The first step in carcinogenesis, whereby limited exposure to a carcinogenic agent produces a latent but heritable alteration in a cell, permitting its subsequent proliferation and development into a neoplasm after exposure to a promoter.

Initiator: A chemical, physical, or biological agent that is capable of irreversibly altering the genetic component (DNA) of the cell. While initiators are generally considered to be carcinogens, they are typically used at low noncarcinogenic doses in two-stage initiation-promotion animal model systems. Frequently referred to as a "tumor initiator."

***In situ* carcinoma**: A localized intraepithelial form of epithelial cell malignancy. The cells possess morphological criteria of malignancy but have not yet gone beyond the limiting basement membrane.

Malignant: A classification of anticipated biological behavior of neoplasms in which the prognosis for survival is poor. Malignant neoplasms grow rapidly, invade, and destroy, and are usually fatal.

Metaplasis: The substitution in a given area of one type of fully differentiated cell for the fully differentiated cell type normally present in that area, e.g. (squamous epithelium replacing ciliated epithelium in the respiratory airways).

Metastasis: The dissemination of cells from a primary neoplasm to a noncontiguous site and their growth therein. Metastases arise by dissemination of cells from the primary neoplasm via the vascular or lymphatic system and are an unequivocal hallmark of malignancy.

Mitogenesis: The generation of cell division or cell proliferation.

MTD (maximum tolerated dose): Refers to the maximum amount of an agent that can be administered to an animal in a carcinogenicity test without adversely affecting the animal due to toxicity other than carcinogenicity. Examples of having exceeded the MTD include excessive early mortality, excessive loss of body weight, production of anemia, production of tissue necrosis, and overloading of the metabolic capacity of the organism.

Mutation: A structural alteration of DNA that is hereditary and gives rise to an abnormal phenotype. A mutation is always a change in the DNA base sequence and includes substitutions, additions, rearrangements, or deletions of one or more nucleotide bases.

Oncogene: The activated form of a protooncogene. Oncogenes are associated with development of neoplasia.

Preneoplastic lesion: A lesion usually indicative that the organism has been exposed to a carcinogen. Presence of preneoplastic lesions indicates that there is enhanced probability for development of neoplasia in the affected organ. Preneoplastic lesions are believed to have a high propensity to progress to neoplasia.

Procarcinogen: An agent that requires bioactivation in order to give rise to a direct-acting carcinogen. Without metabolic activation, these agents are not carcinogenic.

Progression: Processes associated with the development of an initiated cell to a biologically malignant neoplasm. Sometimes used in a more limited sense to describe the process whereby a neoplasm develops from a benign to a malignant proliferation or from a low-grade to a high-grade malignancy. Progression is that stage of neoplastic development characterized by demonstrable changes associated with increased growth rate, increased invasiveness, metastases, and alterations in biochemical and morphologic characteristics of a neoplasm.

Promoter: (1) *Use in multistage carcinogenesis* – an agent that is not carcinogenic itself, but when administered after an initiator of carcinogenesis stimulates the clonal expansion of the initiated cell to produce a neoplasm. (2) *Use in molecular biology* – a DNA sequence that initiates the process of transcription and is located near the beginning of the first exon of a structural gene.

Promotion: The enhancement of neoplasm formation by the administration of a carcinogen, followed by an additional agent (promoter) that has no intrinsic carcinogenic activity by itself.

Protooncogene: A normal cellular structural gene that, when activated by mutations, amplifications, rearrangements, or viral transduction, functions as an oncogene and is associated with development of neoplasia. Protooncogenes regulate functions related to normal growth and differentiation of tissues.

Regulatory gene: A gene that controls the activity of a structural gene or another regulatory gene. Regulatory genes usually do not undergo transcription into messenger RNA.

Sister chromatid exchange: The morphological reflection of an interchange between DNA molecules at homologous loci within a replicating chromosome.

Somatic cell: A normal diploid cell of an organism — as opposed to a germ cell, which is haploid. Most neoplasms are believed to begin when a somatic cell is mutated.

Transformation: Typically refers to tissue culture systems where there is conversion of normal cells into cells with altered phenotypes and growth properties. If such cells are shown to produce invasive neoplasms in animals, malignant transformation is considered to have occurred.

Ultimate carcinogen: That form of the carcinogen that actually interacts with cellular constituents to cause the neoplastic transformation. The final product of metabolism of the procarcinogen.

REPRODUCTIVE/DEVELOPMENTAL TOXICOLOGY

Aberration: A minor structural change. It may be a retardation (a provisional delay in morphogenesis), a variation (external appearance controlled by genetic and extragenetic factors), or a deviation (resulting from altered differentiation).

Ablepharia: Absence or reduction of the eyelid(s).

Abrachius: Without arms, forelimbs.

Acardia: Absence of the heart.

Acaudia (anury): Agenesis of the tail.

Accessory spleen: An additional spleen.

Acephaly: Congenital absence of the head.

Achondroplasia: A hereditary defect in the formation of epiphysial cartilage, resulting in a form of dwarfism with short limbs, normal trunk, small face, normal vault, etc.

Acrania: Partial or complete absence of the skull.

Acystia: Absence of the urinary bladder.

Adactyly: Absence of digits.

Agastria: Absence of the stomach.

Agenesis: Absence of an organ or part of an organ.

Agenesis of the kidney: Absence of the kidney(s).

Agenesis of the lung (lobe): Complete absence of a lobe of the lung.

Aglossia: Absence of the tongue.

Agnathia: Absence of lower jaw (mandible).

Anal atresia: Congenital absence of the anus.

Anencephaly: Congenital absence of the cranial vault with missing or small brain mass.

Anomaly (or abnormality): A morphologic or functional deviation from normal limit; it can be a malformation or a variation.

Anophthalmia: Absence of eye(s).

Anorchism: Congenital absence of one or both testes.

Anotia: Absence of the external ear(s).

Aphalangia: Absence of a finger or a toe; corresponding metacarpals not affected.

Aplasia: Lack of development of an organ, frequently used to designate complete suppression or failure of development of a structure from the embryonic primordium.

Aplasia of the lung: The trachea shows rudimentary bronchi, but pulmonary and vascular structures are absent.

Apodia: Absence of one or both feet.

Aproctia: Imperforation or absence of anus.

Arrhinia: Absence of nose.

Arthrogryposis: Persistent flexure or contracture of a joint; flexed paw (bent at wrist) is most common form of arthrogryposis.

Astomia: Absence of oral orifice.

Brachydactyly: Shortened digits.

Brachyury (short tail): Tail that is reduced in length.

Bulbous rib: Having a bulge or balloon-like enlargement somewhere along its length.

Cardiomegaly: Hypertrophy (enlargement) of the heart.

Cardiovascular situs inversus: Mirror-image transposition of the heart and vessels to the other side of the body.

Cephalocele: A protrusion of a part of the cranial contents, not necessarily neural tissue.

Conceptus: The sum of derivatives of a fertilized ovum at any stage of development from fertilization until birth.

Corpus luteum: The yellow endocrine body formed in the ovary at the site of the ruptured graafian follicle.

Craniorhachischisis: Exencephaly and holorrachischisis (fissure of the spinal cord).

Cranioschisis: Abnormal fissure of the cranium; may be associated with meningocele or encephalocele.

Cryptorchidism (undescended testes, ectopic testes): Failure of the testes to descend into the scrotum (can be unilateral).

Cyclopia: One central orbital fossa with none, one, or two globes.

Deflection: A turning, or state of being turned, aside.

Deformity: Distortion of any part or general disfigurement of the body.

Deviation: Variation from the regular standard or course.

Dextragastria: Having the stomach on the right side of the body.

Dextrocardia: Location of the heart in the right side of the thorax; a developmental disorder associated with total or partial situs inversus (transposition of the great vessels and other thoraco-abdominal organs) or occurs as an isolated anomaly.

Displaced rib: Out of normal position.

Dysgenesis: Defective development; malformation.

Dysmelia: Absence of a portion of one or several limbs.

Dysplasia: (1) Abnormal development of tissues. (2) Alteration in size, shape, or organization of adult cells.

Dystocia: Abnormal labor.

Ectocardia: Displacement of the heart inside or outside the thorax.

Ectopic esophagus: Displacement of the esophagus (description of position should be included).

Ectopic pinna: Displaced external ear.

Ectopic: Out of the normal place.

Ectrodactyly: Absence of all or of only a part of digit (partial ectrodactyly).

Ectromelia: Aplasia or hypoplasia of one or more bones of one or more limbs (this term includes amelia, hemimelia, and phocomelia).

Encephalocele: A partial protrusion of brain through an abnormal cranial opening; not as severe as exencephaly.

Estrus: Phase of the sexual cycle of female mammals, characterized by willingness to mate.

Exencephaly: Brain outside of the skull as a result of a large cranial defect.

Exomphalos: Congenital herniation of abdominal viscera into umbilical cord.

Exophthalmos: Protrusion of the eyeball ("pop" eye).

Fecundity: Ability to produce offspring rapidly and in large numbers.

Feticide: The destruction of the fetus in the uterus.

Gamete: A male (spermatozoon) or female (ovum) reproductive cell.

Gastroschisis: Fissure of abdominal wall (median line) not involving the umbilicus, usually accompanied by protrusion of the small part of the large intestine, not covered by membranous sac.

Hemivertebra: Presence of only one-half of a vertebral body.

Hepatic lobe agenesis: Absence of a lobe of the liver.

Hepatomegaly: Abnormal enlargement of the liver.

Hydrocephaly: Enlargement of the head caused by abnormal accumulation of cerebrospinal fluid in subarachnoid cavity (external hydrocephaly) or ventricular system (internal hydrocephaly).

Hydronephrosis: Dilatation of the renal pelvis, usually combined with destruction of renal parenchyma and often with dilation of the ureters (bilateral, unilateral). *Note*: This is a pathology term and should have histological confirmation.

Hypoplasia of the lung: Bronchial tree poorly developed and pulmonary tissue shows an abnormal histologic picture (total or partial); incomplete development, smaller.

Hypospadias: Urethra opening on the underside of the penis or on the perineum (males), or into the vagina (females).

Imperforate: Not open; abnormally closed.

Incomplete ossification (delayed, retarded): Extent of ossification is less than what would be expected for that developmental age, not necessarily associated with reduced fetal or pup weight.

Levocardia: Displacement of the heart in the extreme left hemithorax.

Lordosis: Anterior concavity in the curvature of the cervical and lumbar spine, as viewed from the side.

Macrobrachia: Abnormal size or length of the arm.

Macrodactylia: Excessive size of one or more digits.

Macroglossia: Enlarged tongue, usually protruding.

Macrophthalmia: Enlarged eye(s).

Meiosis: Cell division occurring in maturation of the sex cell (gametes) by means of which each daughter nucleus receives half the number of chromosomes characteristic of the somatic cells of the species.

Microcephaly: Small head.

Micrognathia: Shortened lower jaw (mandible), tongue may protrude.

Microphthalmia: Small eye(s).

Microstomia: Small mouth opening.

Microtia: Small external ear.

Monocardium: Possessing a heart with only one atrium and one ventricle.

Multigravida: A female pregnant for the second (or more) time.

Naris (nostril) atresia: Absence or closure of nares.

Nasal agenesis: Absence of the nasal cavity and external nose.

Nulliparous: A female that never has born viable offspring.

Oligodactyly: Fewer than normal number of digits.

Oligohydramnios (oligoamnios): Reduction in the amount of amniotic fluid.

Omphalocele: Midline defect in the abdominal wall at the umbilicus, through which the intestines and often other viscera (stomach, spleen, and portions of the liver) protrude. These are always covered by a membranous sac. As a rule, the umbilical cord emerges from the top of the sac.

Pachynsis: Abnormal thickening.

Patent ductus arteriorsus (ductus botalli): An open channel of communication between the main pulmonary artery and the aorta may occur as an isolated abnormality or in combination with other heart defects.

Polydactyly: Extra digits.

Polysomia: A doubling or tripling of the body of a fetus.

Pseudopregnancy: (1) False pregnancy: condition occurring in animals in which anatomical and physiological changes occur similar to those of pregnancy. (2) The premenstrual stage of the endometrium, so-called because it resembles the endometrium just before implantation of the blastocyst.

Rachischisis: Absence of vertebral arches in limited area (partial rachischisis) or entirely (rachischisis totalis).

Renal hypoplasia: Incomplete development of the kidney.

Resorption: A conceptus that, having implanted in the uterus, subsequently died and is being (or has been) resorbed.

Rhinocephaly: A developmental anomaly characterized by the presence of a proboscis-like nose above the eyes, partially or completely fused into one.

Rudimentary rib: Imperfectly developed rib-like structure.

Schistoglossia: Cleft tongue.

Seminiferous epithelium: The normal cellular components within the seminiferous tubule consisting of Sertoli cells, spermatogonia, primary spermatocytes, secondary spermatocytes, and spermatids.

Septal agenesis: Absence of nasal septum.

Sertoli cells: Cells in the testicular tubules providing support, protection, and nutrition for the spermatids.

Spermatocytogenesis: The first stage of spermatogenesis in which spermatogonia develop into spermatocytes and then into spermatids.

Spermiation: The second stage of spermatogenesis, in which the spermatids transform into spermatozoa.

Spina bifida: Defect in closure of bony spinal cavity.

Sympodia: Fusion of the lower extremities.

Syndactyly: Partially or entirely fused digits.

Teratology of fallot: An abnormality of the heart that includes pulmonary stenosis, ventricular septal defect, dextraposition of the aorta overriding the ventricular septum and receiving blood from both ventricles, and right ventricular hypertrophy.

Thoracogastroschisis: Midline fissure in the thorax and abdomen.

Totalis or partialis: Total or partial transposition of viscera (due to incomplete rotation) to the other side of the body; heart most commonly affected (dextrocardia).

Tracheal stenosis: Constriction or narrowing of the tracheal lumen.

Unilobular lung: In the rat fetus, a condition in which the right lung consists of one lobe instead of four separate lobes.

Vaginal plug: A mass of coagulated semen that forms in the vagina of animals after coitus; also called copulation plug or *bouchon vaginal*.

Variation: A minor divergence beyond the usual range of structural constitution.

CLINICAL PATHOLOGY

Activated partial thromboplastin time: A measure of the relative activity of factors in the intrinsic clotting sequence and the common pathway necessary in normal blood coagulation.

Alanine aminotransferase (ALT): An enzyme, primarily of liver origin, whose blood levels can rise in response to hepatocellular toxicity. Also known as SGPT (serum glutamic pyruvic transaminase).

Albumin: The most abundant blood protein synthesized by the liver.

Alkaline phosphatase: An enzyme whose blood levels can rise in response to hepatobiliary disease or increased osteoblastic (bone cell) activity. Serum alkaline phosphatase activity can decrease in fasted rats because the intestinal isozyme is an important component of serum enzyme activity.

Anemia: Any conditions in which RBC count, hemoglobin concentration, and hematocrit are reduced.

Anisocytosis: Variations in the size of red blood cells.

Aspartate aminotransferase (AST): An enzyme whose blood levels can rise in response to hepatotoxicity, muscle damage, or hemolysis. Also known as SGOT (serum glutamic oxaloacetic transaminase).

Azotemia: An increase in serum urea nitrogen and/or creatinine levels.

Creatine kinase (CK): An enzyme that is concentrated in skeletal muscle, brain, and heart tissue.

Creatinine: The end product of creatine metabolism in muscle. Elevated blood levels can indicate renal (glomerular) injury.

Fibrinogen: A glycoprotein that is involved in the formation of fibrin.

Gamma-Glutamyltransferase (γ GT): An enzyme of liver origin, whose blood concentration can be elevated in hepatobiliary disease.

Globulin: A group of blood proteins synthesized by lymphatic tissue in the liver.

Hemolysis: The destruction of red blood cells resulting in liberation of hemoglobin into plasma.

Icteric: Relating to a jaundiced condition, typically as a result of elevated serum bilirubin levels.

Lactate dehydrogenase: An enzyme found in several organs, including liver, kidney, heart, and skeletal muscle.

Mean corpuscular hemoglobin (MCH): The average amount of hemoglobin per red blood cell.

Mean corpuscular hemoglobin concentration (MCHC): The average hemoglobin concentration per red blood cell.

Mean corpuscular volume (MCV): The average size of the red blood cell.

Methemoglobin: Oxidized hemoglobin incapable of carrying oxygen.

Packed cell volume: The percent of blood that contains RBC components; synonymous with hematocrit.

Poikilocytosis: Variations in the shape of red blood cells.

Polychromasia: Increased basophilic staining of erythrocytes.

Polycythemia: An increase in the number of red blood cells.

Prothrombin time: A measure of the relative activity of factors in the extrinsic clotting sequence and the common pathway necessary in normal blood coagulation.

Reticulocyte: An immature (polychromatic) erythrocyte.

Reticulocytosis: Increased numbers of reticulocytes in the circulation, typically seen in response to regenerative anemia.

Sorbitol dehydrogenase (SDH): An enzyme of liver origin, whose blood concentration rises in response to hepatocellular injury.

Triglycerides: Synthesized primarily in the liver and intestine; the major form of lipid storage.

Urea nitrogen (BUN): The end product of protein catabolism. Blood levels can rise after renal (glomerular) injury.

RISK ASSESSMENT: GENERAL

Absorbed dose: The amount of a substance penetrating across the exchange boundaries of an organism and into body fluids and tissues after exposure.

Acceptable daily intake (ADI): A value used for noncarcinogenic effects that represents a daily dose that is very likely to be safe over an extended period of time. An ADI is similar to an RfD (defined below), but less strictly defined.

Administered dose: The amount of a substance given to a human or test animal in determining dose-response relationships, especially through ingestion or inhalation (see applied dose). Administered dose is actually a measure of exposure, because although the substance is "inside" the organism once ingested or inhaled, administered dose does not account for absorption (see absorbed dose).

Aggregate risk: The sum of individual increased risks of an adverse health effect in an exposed population.

Applied dose: The amount of a substance given to a human or test animal in determining dose-response relationships, especially through dermal contact. Applied dose is actually a measure of exposure, since it does not take absorption into account (see absorbed dose).

Biological significant effect: A response in an organism or other biological system that is considered to have a substantial or noteworthy effect (positive or negative) on the well-being of the biological system. Used to distinguish statistically significant effects or changes that may or may not be meaningful to the general state of health of the system.

Cancer potency factor (CPF): The statistical 95% upper confidence limit on the slope of the dose-response relationship at low doses for a carcinogen. Values are in units of lifetime risk per unit dose (mg/kg/day). A plausible upper-bound risk is derived by multiplying the extended lifetime average daily dose (LADD) by the CPF.

Case-control study: A retrospective epidemiological study in which individuals with the disease under study (cases) are compared with individuals without the disease (controls) in order to contrast the extent of exposure in the diseased group with the extent of exposure in the controls.

Ceiling limit: A concentration limit in the workplace that should not be exceeded, even for a short time, to protect workers against frank health effects.

CFR: Code of Federal Regulations.

Cohort study: A study of a group of persons sharing a common experience (e.g., exposure to a substance) within a defined time period; the experiment is used to determine if an increased risk of a health effect (disease) is associated with that exposure.

Confidence limit: The confidence interval is a range of values that has a specified probability (e.g., 95%) of containing a given parameter or characteristic. The confidence limit often refers to the upper value of the range (e.g., upper confidence limit).

Critical endpoint: A chemical may elicit more than one toxic effect (endpoint), even in one test animal, in tests of the same or different duration (acute, subchronic, and chronic exposure studies). The doses that cause these effects may differ. The critical endpoint used in the dose-response assessment is the one that occurs at the lowest dose. In the event that data from multiple species are available, it is often the most sensitive species that determines the critical endpoint. This term is applied in the derivation of risk reference doses.

Cross-sectional study: An epidemiologic study assessing the prevalence of a disease in a population. These studies are most useful for conditions or diseases that are not expected to have a long latent period and do not cause death or withdrawal from the study population. Potential bias in case ascertainment and exposure duration must be addressed when considering cross-sectional studies.

De minimus risk: From the legal maxim *de minimus non curat lex* or the law is not concerned with trifles. As relates to risk assessment of carcinogens, it is commonly interpreted to mean that a lifetime risk of 1×10^{-6} is a **de minimus** level of cancer risk (i.e., insignificant and therefore acceptable) and is of no public health consequence.

Dispersion model: A mathematical model or computer simulation used to predict the movement of airborne or water airborne contaminants. Models take into account a variety of mixing mechanisms which dilute effluents and transport them away from the point of emission.

Dose: The amount of substance administered to an animal or human generally expressed as the weight or volume of the substance per unit of body weight (e.g., mg/kg, ml/kg).

Dose-response relationship: A relationship between (1) the dose, often actually based on "administered dose" (i.e., exposure) rather than absorbed dose, and (2) the extent of toxic injury produced by that chemical. Response can be expressed either as the severity of injury or proportion of exposed subjects affected. A dose-response assessment is one of the steps in a risk assessment.

Duration of exposure: Generally referred to in toxicology as acute (one-time), subacute (repeated over several weeks), subchronic (repeated for a fraction of a lifetime), and chronic (repeated for nearly a lifetime).

Endemic: Present in a community or among a group of people; said of a disease prevailing continually in a region.

Environmental fate: The destiny of a chemical or biological pollutant after release into the environment. Environmental fate involves temporal and spatial considerations of transport, transfer, storage, and transformation.

Exposure: Contact of an organism with a chemical, physical, or biological agent. Exposure is quantified as the amount of the agent available at the exchange boundaries of the organism (e.g., skin, lungs, digestive tract) and available for absorption.

Exposure frequency: The number of times an exposure occurs in a given period. The exposure(s) may be continuous, discontinuous but regular (e.g., once daily), or intermittent.

Extrapolation: An estimate of response or quantity at a point outside the range of the experimental data. Also refers to the estimation of a measured response in a different species or by a different route than that used in the experimental study of interest (i.e., species-to-species, route-to-route, acute-to-chronic, high-to-low).

Fence line concentration: Modeled or measured concentrations of pollutants found at the boundaries of a property on which a pollution source is located. Usually assumed to be the nearest location at which an exposure of the general population could occur.

Frank effect level (FEL): Related to biological responses to chemical exposures (compare with NOAEL and LOEL); the exposure level that produces an unmistakable adverse health effect (such as inflammation, severe convulsions, or death).

Hazard: the inherent ability of a substance to cause an adverse effect under defined conditions of exposure.

Hazard index: the ratio of the maximum daily dose (MDD) to the acceptable daily intake (ADI) used to evaluate the risk of noncarcinogens. A value of less than 1 indicates the risk from the exposure is likely insignificant; a value greater than 1 indicates a potentially significant risk.

Human equivalent dose: The human dose of an agent expected to induce the same type and severity of toxic effect that an animal dose has induced.

Immediately dangerous to life and health (IDLH): A concentration representing the maximum level of a pollutant from which an individual could escape within 30 minutes without escape-impairing symptoms or irreversible health effects.

Incidence: The number of new cases of a disease within a specified time period. It is frequently presented as the number of new cases per 1000, 10,000, or 100,000. The incidence rate is a direct estimate of the probability or risk of developing a disease during a specified time period.

Involuntary risk: A risk that impinges on an individual without his/her awareness or consent.

Latency: The period of time between exposure to an injurious agent and the manifestation of a response.

LC$_{LO}$ (lethal concentration low): The lowest concentration of a chemical required to cause death in some of the population after exposure for a specified period of time and observed for a specified period of time after exposure. Refers to inhalation time exposure in the context of air toxics (may refer to water concentration for tests of aquatic organisms).

LC$_{50}$ (median lethal concentration): The concentration of a chemical required to cause death in 50% of the exposed population when exposed for a specified time period, and observed for a specified period of time after exposure. Refers to inhalation exposure concentration in the context of air toxics (may refer to water concentration for tests of aquatic organisms).

LD$_{LO}$ (lethal dose low): The lowest dose of a chemical required to cause death in some of the population after noninhalation exposure (e.g., injection, ingestion), for a specified observation period after exposure.

LD$_{50}$ (median lethal dose): The dose of a chemical required to cause death in 50% of the exposed population after noninhalation exposure (e.g., injection, ingestion), for a specified observation period after exposure.

Lifetime average daily dose (LADD): The total dose received over a lifetime multiplied by the fraction of a lifetime during which exposure occurs, expressed in mg/kg body weight/day.

Lifetime risk: A risk that results from lifetime exposure.

Lowest-observed-adverse-effect level (LOAEL): The lowest dose or exposure level of a chemical in a study at which there is a statistically or biologically significant increase in the frequency or severity of an *adverse* effect in the exposed population as compared with an appropriate, unexposed control group.

Lowest-observed-effect level (LOEL): In a study, the lowest dose or exposure level of a chemical at which a statistically or biologically significant effect is observed in the exposed population compared with an appropriate unexposed control group. The effect is generally considered not to have an adverse effect on the health and survival of the animal. This term is occasionally misused in place of a LOAEL.

Margin of exposure (MOE): The ratio of the no-observed-adverse-effect level (NOAEL) to the estimated human exposure. The MOE was formerly referred to as the margin of safety (MOS).

Maximum contaminant level (MCL): The maximum level of a contaminant permissible in water as defined by regulations promulgated under the Safety Drinking Water Act.

Maximum daily dose (MDD): Maximum dose received on any given day during a period of exposure, generally expressed in mg/kg body weight/day.

Maximum tolerated dose (MTD): The highest dose of a toxicant that causes toxic effects without causing death during a chronic exposure and that does not decrease the body weight by more than 10%.

Modifying factor (MF): A factor that is greater than zero and less than or equal to 10; it is used in the operational derivation of a reference dose. Its magnitude depends on an assessment of the scientific uncertainties of the toxicological database not explicitly treated with standard uncertainty factors (e.g., number of animals tested). The default value for the MF is 1.

Multistage model: A mathematical function used to extrapolate the probability of incidence of disease from a bioassay in animals using high doses, to that expected to be observed at the low doses that are likely to be found in chronic human exposure. This model is commonly used in quantitative carcinogenic risk assessments where the chemical agent is assumed to be a complete carcinogen and the risk is assumed to be proportional to the dose in the low region.

Nonthreshold toxicant: An agent considered to produce a toxic effect from any dose; any level of exposure is deemed to involve some risk. Usually used only in regard to carcinogenesis.

No-Observed-Adverse-Effect Level (NOAEL): The highest experimental dose at which there is no statistically or biologically significant increase in frequency or severity of *adverse* health effects, as seen in the exposed population compared with an appropriate unexposed population. Effects may be produced at this level, but they are not considered to be adverse.

No-Observed-Effect Level (NOEL): The highest experimental dose at which there is no statistically or biologically significant increase in the frequency or severity of effects seen in the exposed compared with an appropriate unexposed population.

Occupational Exposure Limit (OEL): A generic term denoting a variety of values and standards, generally time-weighted average concentrations of airborne substances to which a worker can be exposed during defined work periods.

Permissible Exposure Limit (PEL): Similar to an occupational exposure limit.

Potency: A comparative expression of chemical or drug activity measured in terms of the relationship between the incidence or intensity of a particular effect and the associated dose of a chemical, to a given or implied standard of reference. Can be used for ranking the toxicity of chemicals.

ppb: Parts per billion.

ppm: Parts per million.

Prevalence: the percentage of a population that is affected with a particular disease at a given time.

q1*: The symbol used to denote the 95% upper bound estimate of the linearized slope of the dose-response curve in the low-dose region as determined by the multistage model.

Reference dose (Rfd): An estimate (with uncertainty spanning perhaps an order of magnitude or more) of the daily exposure to the human population (including sensitive subpopulations) that is likely to be without deleterious effects during a lifetime. The RfD is reported in units of mg of substance/kg body weight/day for oral exposures, or mg/substance/m^3 of air breathed for inhalation exposures (RfC).

Risk: The probability that an adverse effect will occur under a particular condition of exposure.

Risk assessment: The scientific activity of evaluating the toxic properties of a chemical and the conditions of human exposure to it in order to ascertain both the likelihood that exposed humans will be adversely affected, and to characterize the nature of the effects they may experience. May contain some or all of the following four steps.

- **Hazard identification:** The determination of whether a particular chemical is or is not causally linked to particular health effect(s).

- **Dose-response assessment:** The determination of the relation between the magnitude of exposure and the probability of occurrence of the health effects in question.

- **Exposure assessment:** The determination of the extent of human exposure.

- **Risk characterization:** The description of the nature and often the magnitude of human risk, including attendant uncertainty.

Risk management: The decision-making process that uses the results of risk assessment to produce a decision about environmental action. Risk management, includes consideration of technical, scientific, social, economic, and political information.

Short-term exposure limit (STEL): A time-weighted average OEL that the American conference of Government and Industrial Hygienists (ACGIH) indicates should not be exceeded any time during the workday. Exposures at the STEL should not be longer than 15 minutes and should not be repeated more than four (4) times per day. There should be at least 60 minutes between successive exposure at the STEL.

Slope factor: *See* Cancer Potency Factor.

SNUR: Significant New Use Rule.

Standardized mortality ratio: The number of deaths, either total or cause-specific, in a given group expressed as a percentage of the number of deaths that could have been expected if the group has the same age and sex specific rates as the general population. Used in epidemiologic studies to adjust mortality rates to a common standard so that comparisons can be made among groups.

STEL: See short-term exposure limit.

Surface area scaling factor: The intra- and interspecies scaling factor most commonly used for cancer risk assessment by the U.S. EPA to convert an animal dose to a human equivalent dose: milligrams per square meter surface area per day. Body surface area is proportional to basal metabolic rate, the ratio of surface area to metabolic rate tends to be constant from one species to another. Since body surface area is approximately proportional to an animal's body weight to the 2/3 power, the scaling factor can be reduced to (milligrams per body weight)$^{2/3}$.

TC$_{LO}$ (toxic concentration low): The lowest concentration of a substance in air required to cause a toxic effect in some of the exposed population.

TD$_{LO}$ (toxic dose low): The lowest dose of a substance required to cause a toxic effect in some of the exposed population.

Threshold limit value (TLV): The time-weighted average concentration of a substance below which no adverse health effects are expected to occur for workers, assuming exposure for 8 hours per day, 40 hours per week. TLVs are published by the American Conference of Governmental Industrial Hygienists (ACGIH).

Time-weighted average (TWA): An approach to calculating the average exposure over a specified time period.

Uncertainty factor (UF): One of several, generally 10-fold factors, applied to a NOAEL or a LOAEL to derive a reference dose (RfD) from experimental data. UFs are intended to account for (1) the variation in the sensitivity among the members of the human population; (2) the uncertainty in extrapolating animal data to humans; (3) the uncertainty in extrapolating from data obtained in a less-than-lifetime exposure study to chronic exposure; and (4) the uncertainty in using a LOAEL rather than a NOAEL for estimating the threshold region.

Unit cancer risk: A measure of the probability of an individual's developing cancer as a result of exposure to a specified unit ambient concentration. For example, an inhalation unit cancer risk of 3.0×10^{-4} near a point source implies that if 10,000 people breathe a given concentration of a carcinogenic agent (e.g., 1 $\mu g/m^3$) for 70 years, three of the 10,000 will develop cancer as a result of this exposure. In water, the exposure unit is usually 1 µg/l, while in air it is 1 µg/m³).

Upper bound cancer-risk assessment: A qualifying statement indicating that the cancer risk estimate is not a true value, in that the dose-response modeling used provides a value that is not likely to be an underestimate of the true value. The true value may be lower than the upper-bound cancer risk estimate and it may even be close to zero. This results from the use of a statistical upper confidence limit and from the use of conservative assumptions in deriving the cancer risk estimate.

Upper 95% confidence limit: Assuming random and normal distribution, this is the range of values below which a value will fall 95% of the time.

Voluntary risk: Risk that an individual has consciously decided to accept.

References

CARCINOGENESIS:

Maronpot, R.R., *Handbook of Toxicologic Pathology,* Academic Press, San Diego, 1991, 127–129. Reprinted in part with permission.

DERMAL TOXICOLOGY

Cronin, E., *Contact Dermatitis,* Churchill Livingstone, New York, 1980, chaps. 1–17.

Klaassen, C.D., Amdur, M.O., and Doull, J. Eds., *Casarett and Doull's Toxicology, The Basic Science of Poisons,* 4th ed., Pergamon Press, New York, 1991.

Marzulli, F.N. and Maibach, H.I., Eds., *Dermatotoxicology,* 2nd ed., Hemisphere Publishing, Washington, D.C., 1977.

Stedman's Medical Dictionary, 25th ed., Williams & Wilkins, Baltimore, MD, 1990.

Morris, W., Ed., *The American Heritage Dictionary of the English Language, New College Edition*, Houghton Mifflin, Boston, MA., 1978.

United States Environmental Protection Agency, Federal Insecticide, Fungicide, Rodenticide Act, Pesticide Assessment Guidelines, Hazard Evaluation Division, Guidance for Evaluation of Dermal Sensitization, 1, 1984.

REPRODUCTIVE/DEVELOPMENTAL TOXICOLOGY

Middle Atlantic Reproduction and Teratology Association, *A Compilation of Terms Used in Developmental Toxicity Evaluations*, 1989.

RISK ASSESSMENT/GENERAL

Environ Corporation, *Risk Assessment Guidance Manual*, AlliedSignal, Inc., Morristown, NJ, 1990.

United States Environmental Protection Agency, Glossary of Terms Related to Health, Exposure and Risk Assessment, Air Risk Information Support Center, EPA No. 450/3-88/016, 1989.

Balls, M., Blaaboer, B., Brusick, D., Frazier, J., Lamb, D., Pemberton, M., Reinhart, C., Roberfroid, M., Rosenkrantz, H., Schmid, B., Spielmann, H., Stammati, A.-L., and Walum, E., Report and Recommendations of the CAA/ERGATT Workshop on the Validation of Toxicity Test Procedures, ALTA 18, 313, 1990.

Hallenbeck, W.G. and Cunningham, K.M., Eds., *Quantitative Risk Assessment for Environmental and Occupational Health*, Lewis Publishers, Chelsea, MI, 1986, Appendix 2.

Notes